THE MIND DIET FOR SENIORS OVER 60

Delicious Recipes for a Sharper Mind and Vibrant Life.

AISHA D. BASSI

" The Mind Diet for Seniors Over 60: Delicious Recipes for a Sharper Mind and Vibrant Life"

Copyright © 2024 by **Aisha D. Bassi**

Disclaimer:

The information contained in this book is for educational and informational purposes only and is not intended as a substitute for professional advice. The author and publisher shall not be liable for any claims, damages, or losses arising from the use of this book. If you have any concerns about your mental or emotional health, please consult with a qualified professional.

Legal Notice:

Table of Content

Introduction

What is the MIND Diet?

"Let food be thy medicine and medicine be thy food." This ancient wisdom, attributed to Hippocrates, the father of medicine, rings truer than ever as we navigate the complexities of aging. While genetics play a role in our health, research increasingly shows that the foods we choose have a profound impact on our physical and mental well-being, especially as we enter our golden years.

One dietary pattern that has garnered significant attention in recent years is the **MIND diet.** This acronym stands for **Mediterranean-DASH Intervention for Neurodegenerative Delay.** Quite a mouthful, isn't it? But the concept is simple and elegant: By prioritizing specific foods known to support brain health, we can potentially slow cognitive decline and reduce the risk of developing Alzheimer's disease.

The MIND diet is not a fad or a quick fix, but rather a sustainable and enjoyable way of eating that draws inspiration from two well-established diets: the Mediterranean diet and the DASH (Dietary Approaches to Stop Hypertension) diet. These two dietary patterns have been extensively studied and found to have numerous health benefits, including reducing the risk of heart disease, stroke, and type 2 diabetes.

The Mediterranean diet, as the name suggests, is inspired by the traditional eating habits of people living in countries bordering the Mediterranean Sea, such as Greece, Italy, and Spain. It emphasizes whole foods, including fruits, vegetables, whole grains, legumes, nuts, seeds, and olive oil, while limiting processed foods, red meat, and added sugar. The DASH diet, on the other hand, was initially developed to lower blood pressure, but it has since been recognized for its overall health benefits. It emphasizes fruits, vegetables, whole grains, low-fat dairy products, and lean proteins, while limiting sodium, saturated fat, and added sugar.

The MIND diet takes the best aspects of both of these diets and tailors them to specifically target brain health. It emphasizes 10 brain-healthy food groups:

1. **Green leafy vegetables:** Think spinach, kale, collard greens, and other leafy greens. Aim for at least six servings per week. These nutritional powerhouses are packed with vitamins, minerals, and antioxidants that help protect brain cells from damage.

2. **Other vegetables:** In addition to leafy greens, enjoy a variety of colorful vegetables like broccoli, carrots, bell peppers, and onions. Aim for at least one serving per day.

3. **Berries:** Blueberries, strawberries, raspberries, and other berries are rich in antioxidants and anti-inflammatory compounds. Aim for at least two servings per week.

4. **Nuts:** Almonds, walnuts, cashews, and other nuts are excellent sources of healthy fats, protein, and fiber. Aim for at least five servings per week.

5. **Olive oil:** This heart-healthy oil is rich in monounsaturated fats and antioxidants. Use it as your primary cooking oil and for salad dressings.

6. **Whole grains:** Choose whole-wheat bread, brown rice, quinoa, oats, and other whole grains over refined grains. Aim for at least three servings per day.

7. **Fish:** Fatty fish like salmon, tuna, and sardines are rich in omega-3 fatty acids, which are crucial for brain health. Aim for at least one serving per week.

8. **Beans:** Black beans, kidney beans, chickpeas, and other beans are excellent sources of protein, fiber, and other nutrients. Aim for at least three servings per week.

9. **Poultry:** Chicken and turkey are lean sources of protein. Aim for at least two servings per week.

10. **Wine:** While not strictly a food group, moderate wine consumption (one glass per day for women, two for men) has been linked to better cognitive

function in some studies. Choose red wine for its higher antioxidant content.

While the MIND diet encourages the consumption of these 10 brain-healthy food groups, it also recommends limiting the following five unhealthy groups:

1. **Red meat:** Limit red meat consumption to no more than three servings per week.

2. **Butter and stick margarine:** Limit saturated fat from butter and margarine to less than one tablespoon per day.

3. **Cheese:** Limit cheese consumption to no more than one serving per week.

4. **Pastries and sweets:** Limit pastries and sweets to no more than five servings per week.

5. **Fried or fast food:** Limit fried or fast food to less than one serving per week.

The beauty of the MIND diet lies in its flexibility. It's not an all-or-nothing approach, but rather a way of prioritizing certain foods over others.

The Science Behind the MIND Diet

The MIND diet isn't merely a collection of tasty and wholesome foods; it's backed by a growing body of scientific evidence that underscores its potential to safeguard our brains as we age. Numerous studies have explored the link between the MIND diet and cognitive health, revealing promising findings that have captured the attention of researchers, healthcare professionals, and seniors alike.

One of the most compelling studies on the MIND diet was published in 2015 in the journal Alzheimer's & Dementia. This landmark research involved over 900 participants aged 58 to 98 who were followed for an average of 4.5 years. The study found that those who adhered closely to the MIND diet had a 53% lower risk of developing Alzheimer's disease compared to those who did not follow the diet. Even those who moderately adhered to the diet experienced a 35% reduced risk. These results are particularly significant as they suggest that even partial adherence to the MIND diet can confer substantial benefits for brain health.

Another notable study, published in 2023 in the journal Neurology, examined the brains of approximately 600 older adults who had passed away. Through brain autopsies, researchers found that individuals who had reported following the MIND or Mediterranean diet more closely had fewer signs of Alzheimer's disease pathology, including the accumulation of amyloid plaques and tau tangles, which are hallmarks of the disease. This study provided further evidence that the MIND diet may help protect the brain from the damage caused by Alzheimer's.

The mechanisms by which the MIND diet may exert its protective effects on the brain are multifaceted and involve a complex interplay of nutrients and their interactions. While research is ongoing, several key nutrients and their potential mechanisms have emerged as areas of interest:

- **Antioxidants:** Abundant in fruits, vegetables, and berries, antioxidants help neutralize harmful free radicals in the body, which can damage cells and contribute to cognitive decline. Specific antioxidants, such as flavonoids found in berries and vitamin E found in nuts and seeds, have been linked to improved cognitive function and reduced Alzheimer's risk.

- **Omega-3 Fatty Acids:** These essential fats, primarily found in fatty fish like salmon, tuna, and sardines, play a crucial role in brain structure and function. Omega-3s have anti-inflammatory properties and may help protect against age-related cognitive decline and Alzheimer's disease.

- **B Vitamins:** Whole grains, leafy green vegetables, and legumes are rich in B vitamins, particularly folate and vitamin B12, which are essential for maintaining healthy brain cells and neurotransmitters. Deficiencies in these vitamins have been linked to cognitive impairment and an increased risk of Alzheimer's.

- **Vitamin E:** Found in nuts, seeds, and olive oil, vitamin E is a potent antioxidant that may help protect brain cells from damage caused by oxidative stress, a process implicated in Alzheimer's disease.

- **Polyphenols:** These plant compounds, found in fruits, vegetables, and whole grains, have anti-inflammatory and antioxidant properties. They may help protect the brain by reducing inflammation, improving blood flow, and promoting the growth of new brain cells.

The MIND diet's emphasis on whole, unprocessed foods, along with its specific recommendations for brain-healthy nutrients, creates a synergistic effect that goes beyond the benefits of individual nutrients alone. The combined effect of these nutrients, along with the diet's overall emphasis on healthy fats, fiber, and limited processed foods, may help to create an optimal environment for brain health and longevity.

While the research on the MIND diet is still evolving, the existing evidence strongly suggests that this eating pattern holds significant promise for protecting our brains as we age. By making simple, mindful choices about the foods we eat, we can take proactive steps towards maintaining cognitive function and reducing the risk of Alzheimer's disease.

Benefits of the MIND Diet for Seniors

As we journey through life, our bodies undergo natural changes that necessitate a shift in our nutritional priorities. For seniors over 60, maintaining good health and vitality becomes paramount, and the MIND diet emerges as a powerful ally in this endeavor. Tailored to address the unique needs and concerns of aging, this dietary pattern offers a wealth of benefits that extend far beyond brain health.

1. Cardiovascular Health:

Heart disease remains a leading cause of mortality among seniors. The MIND diet, with its emphasis on fruits, vegetables, whole grains, and healthy fats like olive oil, aligns with recommendations for heart health. Studies have shown that adherence to the MIND diet is associated with a reduced risk of cardiovascular events, such as heart attacks and strokes. The abundance of antioxidants and anti-inflammatory compounds in MIND diet foods helps protect blood vessels, lower blood pressure, and improve cholesterol levels, all of which contribute to a healthier heart.

2. Bone Health:

Maintaining strong bones becomes increasingly important as we age, especially for women who are more susceptible to osteoporosis. The MIND diet's inclusion of leafy green vegetables, which are rich in calcium and vitamin K, helps support bone health and may reduce the risk of fractures. Additionally, the diet's emphasis on moderate protein intake from sources like fish, beans, and poultry contributes to bone health without overburdening the kidneys.

3. Gut Health:

A healthy gut microbiome is essential for overall well-being, and its importance only grows with age. The MIND diet's abundance of fiber-rich foods, such as fruits, vegetables, whole grains, and legumes, nourishes beneficial gut bacteria and promotes digestive health. This can help prevent constipation, improve nutrient absorption, and boost the immune system, all of which are vital for seniors.

4. Blood Sugar Control:

Type 2 diabetes is a significant concern for many seniors, but the MIND diet offers a natural way to manage blood sugar levels. The emphasis on whole grains, fruits, and vegetables provides a steady supply of energy without causing spikes in blood sugar. Additionally, the diet's limited intake of added sugars and refined carbohydrates helps prevent insulin resistance and supports stable glucose levels.

5. Weight Management:

Maintaining a healthy weight is crucial for overall health and mobility in older adults. The MIND diet's focus on nutrient-dense, whole foods helps promote satiety and prevent overeating. The high fiber content of the diet also aids in digestion and can contribute to weight loss or maintenance.

6. Eye Health:

Age-related macular degeneration (AMD) is a leading cause of vision loss in seniors. The MIND diet's emphasis on leafy green vegetables, which are rich in lutein and zeaxanthin, may help protect against AMD and preserve vision. Additionally, the diet's inclusion of fish, a good source of omega-3 fatty acids, may also benefit eye health.

7. Reduced Inflammation:

Chronic inflammation is a contributing factor to many age-related diseases, including heart disease, arthritis, and Alzheimer's. The MIND diet's abundance of anti-inflammatory foods, such as berries, leafy greens, and olive oil, helps combat inflammation and protect against its harmful effects.

8. Improved Mood and Mental Well-being:

Emerging research suggests a link between diet and mental health, and the MIND diet may offer a natural way to support emotional well-being in seniors. The diet's rich array of nutrients, including omega-3 fatty acids, B vitamins, and antioxidants, may help reduce the risk of depression and anxiety.

The benefits of the MIND diet for seniors are truly remarkable. By nourishing the body with wholesome foods and limiting those that can harm it, this dietary pattern offers a holistic approach to healthy aging. Whether you're looking to protect your brain, heart, bones, or overall well-being, the MIND diet is a delicious and sustainable way to achieve your health goals and enjoy a vibrant life in your golden years.

Chapter 1: Getting Started with the MIND Diet

Stocking Your MIND Diet Pantry

"Tell me what you eat, and I will tell you who you are." This famous quote by the French gastronome Jean Anthelme Brillat-Savarin speaks to the profound connection between our food choices and our overall well-being. As we embark on the MIND diet journey, transforming our pantry into a haven of brain-healthy foods is a crucial first step.

Imagine your pantry as a well-stocked toolkit, filled with vibrant ingredients ready to nourish your mind and body. Each item you choose is an investment in your long-term health, a building block for delicious meals that not only satisfy your taste buds but also fuel your cognitive vitality.

Let's begin by exploring the foundational elements of your MIND diet pantry, categorized by the essential food groups:

Fruits and Vegetables: A rainbow of colors should fill this section of your pantry. Think leafy greens like spinach, kale, and collard greens, which are packed with vitamins, minerals, and antioxidants that support brain health. Reach for cruciferous vegetables such as broccoli, cauliflower, and Brussels sprouts, known for their anti-inflammatory properties. Don't forget the vibrant hues of bell peppers, carrots, and sweet potatoes, which offer a variety of essential nutrients. And for a burst of flavor and antioxidants, stock up on berries – blueberries, strawberries, raspberries, and blackberries are all excellent choices.

Tips:

- Choose seasonal produce whenever possible. It's not only fresher and more flavorful, but it's also often more affordable.

- Look for locally grown options at farmers markets or community-supported agriculture (CSA) programs. This supports local farmers and reduces the environmental impact of transporting food over long distances.

- Frozen fruits and vegetables can be a convenient and budget-friendly alternative to fresh produce. They're often picked at peak ripeness and flash-frozen to preserve nutrients.

- Consider growing your own herbs and vegetables if you have the space and time. It's a rewarding way to enjoy fresh, organic produce.

Whole Grains: Whole grains are the backbone of a healthy diet, providing sustained energy, fiber, and essential nutrients. Opt for whole-wheat bread, brown rice, quinoa, oats, farro, and barley over their refined counterparts. These complex carbohydrates are digested slowly, helping to stabilize blood sugar levels and promote satiety.

Tips:

- Look for whole-grain products that list whole wheat, brown rice, oats, or another whole grain as the first ingredient.

- Experiment with different types of whole grains to add variety to your meals.

- Cook a large batch of whole grains at the beginning of the week and store them in the refrigerator or freezer for easy access.

Legumes: Beans, lentils, and chickpeas are nutritional powerhouses, packed with protein, fiber, and iron. They're also incredibly versatile and can be used in soups, stews, salads, and main dishes. Dried beans and lentils are a budget-friendly option, but canned varieties are convenient when you're short on time.

Tips:

- Rinse canned beans thoroughly to reduce sodium content.

- Soak dried beans overnight to reduce cooking time and improve digestibility.

- Cook a large batch of beans or lentils and freeze them in portion sizes for future meals.

Nuts and Seeds: Almonds, walnuts, cashews, sunflower seeds, pumpkin seeds, and flaxseeds are all excellent sources of healthy fats, protein, and fiber. Enjoy them as a snack, sprinkle them on salads or yogurt, or add them to baked goods.

Tips:

- Buy nuts and seeds in bulk to save money.

- Store them in airtight containers in a cool, dark place to preserve freshness.

Olive Oil: This heart-healthy oil is the cornerstone of the Mediterranean diet and a staple in the MIND diet. It's rich in monounsaturated fats, which can help lower bad cholesterol levels and reduce the risk of heart disease. Use extra-virgin olive oil for salad dressings and drizzling over finished dishes, and regular olive oil for cooking.

Tips:

- Look for olive oil that is labeled "extra-virgin" and cold-pressed for the highest quality.

- Store olive oil in a cool, dark place to protect it from light and heat, which can degrade its flavor and nutritional value.

Fish: Fatty fish like salmon, tuna, sardines, and mackerel are rich in omega-3 fatty acids, which are essential for brain health. Aim to include at least two servings of fish per week in your diet.

Tips:

- Choose wild-caught fish whenever possible to reduce exposure to contaminants.

- Fresh fish is ideal, but frozen or canned varieties can be convenient options.

- If you're not a fan of fish, consider taking a fish oil supplement to ensure you're getting enough omega-3s.

Poultry: Chicken and turkey are lean sources of protein that can be incorporated into a variety of dishes. Choose skinless, boneless breasts or thighs to minimize saturated fat intake.

Tips:

- Buy whole chickens or turkeys and learn to butcher them yourself to save money.

- Roast a whole chicken or turkey at the beginning of the week and use the leftovers in salads, sandwiches, and other dishes.

- Marinate chicken or turkey breasts before grilling or baking to enhance flavor and tenderness.

Dairy: Low-fat dairy products like milk, yogurt, and cheese can be part of the MIND diet in moderation. Choose options that are fortified with vitamin D, which is essential for bone health and calcium absorption.

Tips:

- Greek yogurt is a good source of protein and probiotics, which are beneficial for gut health.

- Look for cheese varieties that are lower in sodium and saturated fat, such as mozzarella, feta, or cottage cheese.

Eggs: Eggs are a versatile source of protein and nutrients like choline, which is important for brain health. They can be enjoyed for breakfast, lunch, or dinner.

Tips:

- Choose organic, free-range eggs whenever possible.

- Experiment with different cooking methods, such as poaching, scrambling, or hard-boiling.

Herbs and Spices: Not only do herbs and spices add flavor and depth to your dishes, but they also offer a range of health benefits. Turmeric, ginger, garlic, and cinnamon all have anti-inflammatory properties, while rosemary and sage have been linked to improved memory and cognitive function.

Tips:

- Buy fresh herbs whenever possible and store them in a jar of water in the refrigerator.

- Create your own spice blends to add a unique touch to your meals.

Other Pantry Staples:

- **Vinegar:** Balsamic vinegar, apple cider vinegar, and red wine vinegar can be used to make salad dressings, marinades, and sauces.

- **Honey or Maple Syrup:** Use these natural sweeteners in moderation to add a touch of sweetness to smoothies, yogurt, or oatmeal.

- **Whole-Wheat Flour:** Use this for baking bread, muffins, and other baked goods.

- **Brown Rice:** This versatile grain can be used in salads, stir-fries, and as a side dish.

- **Quinoa:** This ancient grain is a complete protein and a good source of fiber. It can be used in place of rice or couscous.

- **Oats:** Oats are a hearty and nutritious breakfast option. They can also be used in baked goods or added to smoothies.

By stocking your pantry with these nutritious staples, you'll be well on your way to embracing the MIND diet and enjoying its many benefits for your brain and overall health. Remember, the key is to focus on whole, unprocessed foods that are packed with nutrients and flavor. With a little creativity and planning, you can easily transform these simple ingredients into delicious and satisfying meals that nourish your body and mind.

As you explore the recipes in this book, you'll find countless ways to incorporate these pantry staples into your daily meals. From hearty lentil stews and vibrant salads to flavorful fish dishes and satisfying snacks, the MIND diet offers a wealth of culinary possibilities.

Essential MIND Diet Cooking Tips

In the kitchen, as in life, simple pleasures often yield the most rewarding results. The MIND diet is a testament to this philosophy, emphasizing wholesome ingredients and straightforward cooking techniques that enhance both flavor and nutrition. For seniors, this approach is particularly appealing, offering a path to delicious, brain-boosting meals without the need for elaborate recipes or hours spent in the kitchen.

Let's explore some essential cooking tips that will elevate your MIND diet experience and empower you to create meals that are both satisfying and nourishing. We'll focus on techniques that maximize flavor, preserve nutrients, and simplify your time in the kitchen.

Roasting Vegetables:

Roasting is a simple yet transformative technique that brings out the natural sweetness and complexity of vegetables. The high heat caramelizes their sugars, creating a depth of flavor that is both savory and satisfying. To roast vegetables, toss them with olive oil, salt, pepper, and your favorite herbs and spices. Spread them in a single layer on a baking sheet and roast in a preheated oven until tender and slightly browned.

- **Recipe Idea:** Roasted Root Vegetables with Rosemary and Garlic: This easy recipe combines carrots, parsnips, sweet potatoes, and onions, roasted with fragrant rosemary and garlic. It's a perfect side dish or can be enjoyed as a light meal.

Grilling Fish:

Grilling imparts a smoky flavor to fish while keeping it moist and tender. To grill fish, brush it with olive oil and season it with salt, pepper, and herbs. Cook it over medium heat until it is opaque and flakes easily with a fork. Grilling is also a great way to cook vegetables, such as zucchini, eggplant, and bell peppers.

- **Recipe Idea:** Grilled Salmon with Lemon-Dill Sauce: This simple yet elegant dish features salmon fillets grilled to perfection and topped with a refreshing lemon-dill sauce. Serve it with a side of roasted vegetables or a quinoa salad for a complete meal.

Sautéing Greens:

Leafy greens, such as spinach, kale, and collard greens, are nutritional powerhouses, but they can be tricky to cook. Sautéing them quickly in olive oil with garlic and a pinch of red pepper flakes helps to soften them and enhance their flavor. You can also add a splash of lemon juice or balsamic vinegar at the end for extra brightness.

- **Recipe Idea:** Sautéed Kale with Garlic and Lemon: This quick and easy side dish is packed with nutrients and flavor. It's a great way to add more leafy greens to your diet.

One-Pan Meals:

One-pan meals are a lifesaver for busy weeknights. They require minimal prep time and cleanup, making them ideal for seniors who want to spend less time in the kitchen. To create a one-pan meal, simply combine your protein of choice (chicken, fish, tofu, or beans) with vegetables and a flavorful sauce on a baking sheet or in a skillet. Bake or cook on the stovetop until everything is cooked through.

- **Recipe Idea:** One-Pan Lemon Herb Chicken and Vegetables: This simple recipe features chicken breasts, potatoes, carrots, and broccoli, all cooked together on a sheet pan with lemon, herbs, and olive oil. It's a complete meal that's ready in under an hour.

Sheet-Pan Dinners:

Similar to one-pan meals, sheet-pan dinners offer convenience and ease. They're perfect for cooking larger batches of food, which can be enjoyed for leftovers throughout the week. To create a sheet-pan dinner, simply spread your protein and vegetables in a single layer on a baking sheet, drizzle with olive oil, season with salt, pepper, and herbs, and roast in a preheated oven until everything is tender and cooked through.

- **Recipe Idea:** Sheet-Pan Salmon with Roasted Vegetables: This healthy and flavorful dish features salmon fillets, asparagus, Brussels sprouts, and sweet potatoes, all roasted together on a sheet pan with lemon, garlic, and olive oil.

Slow-Cooker Meals:

Slow cookers are a fantastic tool for seniors who want to come home to a warm and comforting meal without having to spend hours in the kitchen. Simply add your ingredients to the slow cooker in the morning, set it, and forget it. By dinnertime, you'll have a delicious and nutritious meal that's ready to enjoy.

- **Recipe Idea:** Slow-Cooker Lentil Soup: This hearty and flavorful soup is packed with protein, fiber, and nutrients. It's a perfect meal for a cold winter day and can be easily frozen for later.

Beyond these fundamental techniques, a few additional tips can further enhance your MIND diet cooking experience:

Flavorful Sauces and Dressings:

Homemade sauces and dressings are a simple way to elevate the flavor of your meals while adding extra nutrients and antioxidants. Instead of relying on store-bought options, which can be high in sodium, sugar, and unhealthy fats, experiment with creating your own using olive oil, vinegar, herbs, spices, and other MIND-approved ingredients.

- **Recipe Idea:** Lemon-Tahini Dressing: This creamy and tangy dressing is made with tahini, lemon juice, olive oil, garlic, and a touch of honey. It's perfect for drizzling over salads or roasted vegetables.

Batch Cooking:

Prepare larger batches of grains, beans, and roasted vegetables at the beginning of the week. This will save you time and effort on busy days, ensuring you have healthy ingredients on hand to quickly assemble meals. You can also portion out individual servings and freeze them for later.

- **Recipe Idea:** Quinoa and Black Bean Salad: This versatile salad can be made ahead of time and enjoyed throughout the week. It's packed with protein, fiber, and flavor, making it a satisfying and nutritious meal.

Use Fresh Herbs:

Fresh herbs add a burst of flavor and freshness to any dish. They're also packed with antioxidants and other beneficial compounds. Grow your own herbs or purchase them from the grocery store and use them generously in your cooking.

- **Recipe Idea:** Herbed Chicken Breast: This simple recipe features chicken breasts seasoned with a blend of fresh herbs, such as rosemary, thyme, and oregano. It's a light and flavorful dish that's perfect for a weeknight meal.

Don't Be Afraid to Experiment:

The MIND diet is not about strict rules or deprivation; it's about enjoying a variety of delicious and nutritious foods. Feel free to experiment with different ingredients and flavor combinations to find what you enjoy most. The most important thing is to focus on whole, unprocessed foods that are good for your body and your brain.

- **Recipe Idea:** Mediterranean Veggie Bowl: This customizable bowl is a great way to use up leftover vegetables and grains. Simply combine your favorite roasted vegetables, cooked grains, beans, and a dollop of hummus or tahini sauce.

Additional Tips for Seniors:

- **Make it Social:** Invite friends or family over for a cooking session or potluck. Cooking and eating together can be a fun and social way to enjoy the MIND diet.

- **Keep it Simple:** Don't feel pressured to cook elaborate meals every day. Simple, healthy dishes can be just as satisfying.

- **Modify as Needed:** If you have dietary restrictions or preferences, feel free to modify recipes to suit your needs.

- **Seek Inspiration:** Look for cookbooks, websites, and blogs that offer MIND diet-friendly recipes. There are countless delicious and healthy options to explore.

By incorporating these essential cooking tips into your routine, you can make the MIND diet a sustainable and enjoyable part of your lifestyle. Remember, healthy eating doesn't have to be complicated or time-consuming. With a few simple techniques and a focus on whole, unprocessed foods, you can create delicious meals that nourish your body and mind.

As you embark on this culinary adventure, remember to savor each bite and appreciate the vibrant flavors and textures of the MIND diet. Let food be your ally in maintaining a healthy brain and a fulfilling life.

Navigating Dining Out and Special Occasions

While the comfort and control of your own kitchen provide an ideal environment for embracing the MIND diet, life inevitably presents situations where dining out or attending social gatherings is unavoidable. However, these occasions need not derail your commitment to healthy eating. With a bit of knowledge and preparation, you can navigate restaurant menus and social events while staying true to the principles of the MIND diet.

Let's delve into some practical strategies for making mindful choices and enjoying the social aspects of dining without compromising your nutritional goals.

Before You Go:

Planning is key when it comes to dining out on the MIND diet. A little research can go a long way in ensuring a satisfying and healthy experience.

- **Check the Menu Online:** Most restaurants have their menus available online. Take some time to review the options beforehand and identify dishes that align with the MIND diet principles. Look for items that feature grilled or baked fish, chicken, or tofu, as well as salads, vegetable-based sides, and whole-grain options.

- **Have a Plan:** Decide what you'll order before you arrive at the restaurant. This will help you avoid impulsive choices and stay focused on your health goals.

- **Communicate Your Needs:** Don't be afraid to ask questions about ingredients, preparation methods, and portion sizes. Most restaurants are happy to accommodate special requests.

At the Restaurant:

- **Start with a Salad:** A salad is a great way to fill up on vegetables and fiber, which can help you feel satisfied and prevent overeating. Choose a salad with leafy greens, vegetables, and a vinaigrette dressing made with olive oil.

- **Choose Grilled or Baked Dishes:** These cooking methods are healthier than frying and can be used to prepare a variety of MIND-friendly proteins, such as fish, chicken, or tofu.

- **Ask for Modifications:** Don't hesitate to ask for substitutions or modifications to make a dish more MIND-friendly. For example, you could ask for a side of vegetables instead of fries, or request that your meal be prepared with olive oil instead of butter.

- **Practice Portion Control:** Restaurant portions are often larger than necessary. Consider sharing a meal with a friend or taking half of your meal home for later.

- **Be Mindful of Sauces and Dressings:** These can add a lot of extra calories, sodium, and unhealthy fats to your meal. Ask for sauces and dressings on the side so you can control how much you use.

Social Gatherings:

Social gatherings can present a challenge for those following the MIND diet, but with a bit of creativity and flexibility, you can still enjoy the festivities while making healthy choices.

- **Offer to Bring a Dish:** If you're attending a potluck or party, offer to bring a MIND-friendly dish to share. This way, you'll know there's at least one healthy option available.

- **Fill Up on Vegetables:** Before you reach for the chips and dip, fill your plate with vegetables and fruits. This will help you feel satisfied and prevent overeating later.

- **Choose Mindful Indulgences:** It's okay to indulge in a small treat or a glass of wine, but try to be mindful of your choices and enjoy them in moderation.

- **Focus on Socializing:** Remember that social gatherings are about connecting with others, not just about the food. Focus on conversations and activities, and don't let food become the center of attention.

Tips for Dining Out on a Budget:

- **Lunch Specials:** Many restaurants offer lunch specials that are more affordable than dinner entrees.

- **Early Bird Specials:** Some restaurants offer discounts for early diners.

- **Happy Hour:** Appetizers and drinks are often discounted during happy hour.

- **BYOB:** If you enjoy wine, consider bringing your own bottle to a restaurant that allows it. This can save you money on alcohol.

- **Split a Meal:** Share a meal with a friend or family member to cut costs.

With these strategies in your arsenal, you can confidently navigate dining out and special occasions while staying true to your MIND diet goals. Remember, the MIND diet is not about deprivation or restriction; it's about making informed choices and enjoying the pleasures of food while nourishing your body and brain.

By prioritizing whole, unprocessed foods, practicing portion control, and making mindful substitutions, you can easily incorporate the MIND diet into your social life without feeling like you're missing out. Remember, it's about finding a balance that works for you and enjoying the journey of healthy eating.

As you venture out to restaurants and social gatherings, keep in mind that the MIND diet is a lifestyle, not a rigid set of rules. Be flexible, adaptable, and most importantly, enjoy the experience of sharing meals with loved ones and savoring the flavors of delicious and nutritious food.

Chapter 2: Smoothies and Breakfast

"Breakfast is everything. The beginning, the first thing. It is the mouthful that is the commitment to a new day, a continuing life." A.A. Gill's words ring true, emphasizing the importance of starting our day with nourishment. For seniors, a MIND diet-approved breakfast is not just a meal; it's a foundation for cognitive vitality, energy, and overall well-being.

This chapter is your gateway to a world of flavorful and brain-boosting breakfast options, each designed to tantalize your taste buds and fuel your day. From refreshing smoothies bursting with antioxidants to savory egg dishes packed with protein, you'll find a diverse range of recipes to suit your preferences and dietary needs.

Let's embark on a culinary journey through 20 unique breakfast recipes that celebrate the MIND diet's principles of wholesome ingredients, vibrant flavors, and effortless preparation.

1. Berry Blast Smoothie

Servings: 1   **Prep time:** 5 minutes

Ingredients:

- 1 cup frozen mixed berries (blueberries, strawberries, raspberries)

- ½ cup plain Greek yogurt

- ½ cup almond milk (or other milk of choice)

- 1 tablespoon chia seeds

- ½ banana, frozen

Instructions:

1. Combine all ingredients in a blender.

2. Blend until smooth and creamy.

3. Pour into a glass and enjoy immediately.

Nutritional Information: Calories: 250, Protein: 12g, Fat: 6g, Fiber: 8g

2. Tropical Green Smoothie
Servings: *1* ***Prep time:*** *5 minutes*

Ingredients:

- 1 cup chopped kale or spinach

- ½ cup chopped pineapple

- ½ cup chopped mango

- ½ cup coconut water

- ½ banana, frozen

Instructions:

1. Combine all ingredients in a blender.

2. Blend until smooth and creamy.

3. Pour into a glass and enjoy immediately.

Nutritional Information: *Calories: 230, Protein: 4g, Fat: 3g, Fiber: 6g*

3. Savory Oatmeal with Spinach and Egg

Servings: *1* ***Prep time:*** *10 minutes*

Ingredients:

- ½ cup rolled oats
- 1 cup water
- ¼ teaspoon salt
- ½ cup chopped spinach
- 1 egg
- Pinch of black pepper

Instructions:

1. Combine oats, water, and salt in a saucepan.
2. Bring to a boil, then reduce heat and simmer for 5 minutes, or until oats are cooked through.
3. While oats are cooking, fry the egg in a separate pan.
4. Stir spinach into the cooked oatmeal.
5. Top with the fried egg and a pinch of black pepper.

Nutritional Information: *Calories: 280, Protein: 15g, Fat: 9g, Fiber: 7g*

4. Avocado Toast with Tomato and Feta

Servings: *1* ***Prep time:*** *5 minutes*

Ingredients:

- 1 slice whole-wheat bread, toasted

- ½ avocado, mashed

- ¼ cup chopped tomato

- 1 tablespoon crumbled feta cheese

- Pinch of red pepper flakes

Instructions:

1. Spread mashed avocado on toast.

2. Top with chopped tomato and feta cheese.

3. Sprinkle with red pepper flakes.

Nutritional Information: *Calories: 300, Protein: 10g, Fat: 18g, Fiber: 8g*

5. Berry Parfait with Granola and Nuts

Servings: 1   **Prep time:** 5 minutes

Ingredients:

- ½ cup plain Greek yogurt

- ½ cup mixed berries

- ¼ cup granola

- 1 tablespoon chopped nuts (almonds, walnuts, or pecans)

Instructions:

1. Layer yogurt, berries, granola, and nuts in a glass or bowl.

2. Repeat layers as desired.

3. Enjoy immediately.

Nutritional Information: *Calories: 350, Protein: 14g, Fat: 16g, Fiber: 8g*

6. Spinach and Feta Frittata

Servings: *2* **Prep time:** *15 minutes*

Ingredients:

- 4 eggs
- ½ cup chopped spinach
- ¼ cup crumbled feta cheese
- 1 tablespoon olive oil
- Salt and pepper to taste

Instructions:

1. Preheat oven to 350°F (175°C).
2. Whisk eggs, spinach, feta, salt, and pepper in a bowl.
3. Heat olive oil in an oven-safe skillet over medium heat.
4. Pour egg mixture into the skillet and cook for 2-3 minutes, or until the edges are set.
5. Transfer skillet to the oven and bake for 10-12 minutes, or until the frittata is set in the center.
6. Let cool slightly before cutting into wedges and serving.

Nutritional Information (per serving): *Calories: 200, Protein: 14g, Fat: 14g, Fiber: 1g*

7. Berry Chia Seed Pudding

Servings: *1* ***Prep time:*** *5 minutes (plus overnight chilling)*

Ingredients:

- ¼ cup chia seeds
- 1 cup almond milk (or other milk of choice)
- 2 tablespoons maple syrup or honey
- ½ teaspoon vanilla extract
- ½ cup mixed berries

Instructions:

1. In a jar or bowl, combine chia seeds, milk, maple syrup/honey, and vanilla extract.
2. Stir well to combine and let sit for 5 minutes, then stir again to prevent clumping.
3. Refrigerate overnight (or for at least 4 hours) until pudding thickens.
4. Top with mixed berries before serving.

Nutritional Information: *Calories: 250, Protein: 6g, Fat: 11g, Fiber: 15g*

8. Banana Nut Oatmeal

Servings: *1* ***Prep time:*** *5 minutes*

Ingredients:

- ½ cup rolled oats
- 1 cup water or milk of choice
- Pinch of salt
- ½ banana, sliced
- 1 tablespoon chopped nuts (almonds, walnuts, or pecans)
- Drizzle of honey or maple syrup (optional)

Instructions:

1. Combine oats, water/milk, and salt in a saucepan.
2. Bring to a boil, then reduce heat and simmer for 5 minutes, or until oats are cooked through.
3. Top with sliced banana, chopped nuts, and a drizzle of honey or maple syrup (if desired).

Nutritional Information: *Calories: 250, Protein: 8g, Fat: 7g, Fiber: 8g*

9. Whole-Wheat Pancakes with Berries

Servings: *2* ***Prep time:*** *15 minutes*

Ingredients:

- 1 cup whole-wheat flour
- 2 teaspoons baking powder
- ½ teaspoon baking soda
- ¼ teaspoon salt
- 1 egg
- 1 cup milk of choice
- 1 tablespoon olive oil
- ½ cup mixed berries

Instructions:

1. In a bowl, whisk together flour, baking powder, baking soda, and salt.
2. In a separate bowl, whisk together egg, milk, and olive oil.
3. Pour wet ingredients into dry ingredients and stir until just combined (batter will be slightly lumpy).
4. Heat a lightly oiled griddle or frying pan over medium heat.
5. Pour ¼ cup of batter onto the griddle for each pancake.

6. Cook for 2-3 minutes per side, or until golden brown and cooked through.

7. Serve warm with berries.

Nutritional Information (per serving): *Calories: 280, Protein: 10g, Fat: 10g, Fiber: 6g*

10. Mediterranean Egg Scramble

Servings: *1* **Prep time:** *10 minutes*

Ingredients:

- 2 eggs
- ¼ cup chopped onion
- ¼ cup chopped bell pepper
- ¼ cup chopped tomato
- 1 tablespoon olive oil
- Pinch of salt and pepper
- ½ ounce crumbled feta cheese

Instructions:

1. Heat olive oil in a pan over medium heat.
2. Add onion and bell pepper and cook for 3-4 minutes, or until softened.
3. Add tomato and cook for another 1-2 minutes.
4. Beat eggs in a bowl and season with salt and pepper.
5. Pour eggs into the pan and scramble until cooked through.
6. Sprinkle with feta cheese before serving.

Nutritional Information: *Calories: 250, Protein: 15g, Fat: 18g, Fiber: 2g*

11. Tofu Scramble with Spinach and Tomatoes

Servings: *1* ***Prep time:*** *15 minutes*

Ingredients:

- ½ block firm tofu, crumbled
- ½ cup chopped spinach
- ¼ cup chopped tomatoes
- 1 tablespoon olive oil
- ½ teaspoon turmeric
- ½ teaspoon cumin
- Pinch of salt and pepper

Instructions:

1. Heat olive oil in a pan over medium heat.
2. Add tofu and cook for 5-7 minutes, or until lightly browned.
3. Add spinach, tomatoes, turmeric, cumin, salt, and pepper.
4. Cook for another 3-4 minutes, or until spinach is wilted and tomatoes are softened.

Nutritional Information: *Calories: 280, Protein: 18g, Fat: 16g, Fiber: 5g*

12. Lemony Yogurt with Berries and Granola

Servings: 1 Prep time: 5 minutes

Ingredients:

- ½ cup plain Greek yogurt

- 1 tablespoon honey or maple syrup

- ½ teaspoon lemon zest

- ¼ cup mixed berries

- ¼ cup granola

Instructions:

1. In a bowl, combine yogurt, honey/maple syrup, and lemon zest.

2. Top with berries and granola.

Nutritional Information: *Calories: 270, Protein: 12g, Fat: 8g, Fiber: 6g*

13. Apple Cinnamon Baked Oatmeal

Servings: *2* ***Prep time:*** *10 minutes (plus 30 minutes baking time)*

Ingredients:

- 1 cup rolled oats
- 1 ½ cups milk of choice
- 1 apple, chopped
- ½ teaspoon cinnamon
- Pinch of salt
- 2 tablespoons chopped nuts (optional)

Instructions:

1. Preheat oven to 375°F (190°C).
2. Combine oats, milk, apple, cinnamon, and salt in a baking dish.
3. Stir to combine.
4. Bake for 30 minutes, or until golden brown and set.
5. Top with chopped nuts (optional) before serving.

Nutritional Information (per serving): *Calories: 240, Protein: 8g, Fat: 8g, Fiber: 8g*

14. Sweet Potato and Black Bean Hash

***Servings:** 2 **Prep time:** 20 minutes*

Ingredients:

- 1 tablespoon olive oil
- 1 sweet potato, diced
- ½ onion, chopped
- 1 can black beans, rinsed and drained
- 1 bell pepper, chopped
- ½ teaspoon chili powder
- ½ teaspoon cumin
- Salt and pepper to taste
- 2 eggs (optional)

1. Heat olive oil in a pan over medium heat.
2. Add sweet potato and onion and cook for 5-7 minutes, or until softened.
3. Add black beans, bell pepper, chili powder, cumin, salt, and pepper.
4. Cook for another 5-7 minutes, or until heated through.
5. If desired, fry two eggs in a separate pan and serve on top of the hash.

Nutritional Information (per serving without egg): *Calories: 300, Protein: 12g, Fat: 9g, Fiber: 15g*

15. Smoked Salmon and Cream Cheese Egg Wraps

Servings: *1* ***Prep time:*** *5 minutes*

Ingredients:

- 2 eggs
- 1 tablespoon cream cheese
- 1-ounce smoked salmon
- 1 tablespoon chopped chives
- Salt and pepper to taste

Instructions:

1. Whisk eggs in a bowl and season with salt and pepper.
2. Heat a lightly oiled pan over medium heat.
3. Pour eggs into the pan and cook for 2-3 minutes, or until set.
4. Spread cream cheese over the egg wrap.
5. Top with smoked salmon and chives.
6. Roll up and enjoy.

Nutritional Information: *Calories: 350, Protein: 20g, Fat: 25g, Fiber: 1g*

16. Mediterranean Chickpea Salad

Servings: 2 **Prep time:** *15 minutes*

Ingredients:

- 1 can chickpeas, rinsed and drained
- ½ cup chopped cucumber
- ½ cup chopped tomato
- ¼ cup chopped red onion
- ¼ cup chopped Kalamata olives
- 2 tablespoons chopped fresh parsley
- 2 tablespoons lemon juice
- 2 tablespoons olive oil
- Salt and pepper to taste

Instructions:

1. Combine all ingredients in a bowl.
2. Stir to combine.
3. Serve chilled or at room temperature.

Nutritional Information (per serving): *Calories: 250, Protein: 10g, Fat: 12g, Fiber: 10g*

17. Whole-Wheat Toast with Almond Butter and Banana

Servings: *1* ***Prep time:*** *5 minutes*

Ingredients:

- 1 slice whole-wheat bread, toasted

- 1 tablespoon almond butter

- ½ banana, sliced

Instructions:

1. Spread almond butter on toast.

2. Top with sliced banana.

Nutritional Information: *Calories: 220, Protein: 8g, Fat: 10g, Fiber: 5g*

18. Cottage Cheese with Berries and Nuts

Servings: *1* ***Prep time:*** *5 minutes*

Ingredients:

- ½ cup cottage cheese

- ½ cup mixed berries

- 1 tablespoon chopped nuts (almonds, walnuts, or pecans)

Instructions:

1. Top cottage cheese with berries and nuts.

Nutritional Information: *Calories: 200, Protein: 18g, Fat: 8g, Fiber: 4g*

19. Greek Yogurt with Honey and Fruit

Servings: *1* **Prep time:** *5 minutes*

Ingredients:

- ½ cup plain Greek yogurt

- 1 tablespoon honey

- ½ cup chopped fruit (berries, banana, or peaches)

Instructions:

1. Combine yogurt and honey.

2. Top with chopped fruit.

Nutritional Information: *Calories: 200, Protein: 14g, Fat: 4g, Fiber: 4g*

20. Quinoa Breakfast Bowl

Servings: *1* **Prep time:** *15 minutes*

Ingredients:

- ½ cup cooked quinoa

- ½ cup milk of choice

- ½ teaspoon cinnamon

- Pinch of salt

- ½ cup mixed berries

- 1 tablespoon chopped nuts (almonds, walnuts, or pecans)

Instructions:

1. Combine quinoa, milk, cinnamon, and salt in a saucepan.

2. Heat over medium heat until warm.

3. Top with berries and nuts.

Nutritional Information: *Calories: 300, Protein: 10g, Fat: 10g, Fiber: 8g*

The MIND diet doesn't limit you to bland or boring breakfasts. With a little creativity, you can enjoy a wide variety of flavorful and nutritious meals that nourish your body and brain. These recipes are just a starting point – feel free to experiment with different ingredients and combinations to find what you enjoy most.

Chapter 3: Salads, Soups, and Sides

"A salad is not a meal, it is a style." This witty remark by American chef and author David Lebovitz rings true in the context of the MIND diet. Salads, soups, and sides aren't mere accompaniments; they are the vibrant canvases upon which we paint a picture of health and flavor. These dishes, bursting with colorful vegetables, legumes, whole grains, and healthy fats, are the unsung heroes of the MIND diet, providing essential nutrients and antioxidants that nourish our bodies and brains.

In this chapter, we invite you to explore the delightful world of salads, soups, and sides, where creativity and nourishment intertwine. You'll discover 20 unique recipes that celebrate the MIND diet's principles of wholesome ingredients, diverse flavors, and effortless preparation. Whether you're seeking a light lunch, a satisfying side dish, or a comforting bowl of soup, you'll find an abundance of options to tantalize your taste buds and fuel your well-being.

1. Mediterranean Chickpea Salad

Servings: *2* ***Prep time:*** *15 minutes*

Ingredients:

- 1 can (15 ounces) chickpeas, rinsed and drained
- 1 cup chopped cucumber
- 1 cup chopped tomatoes
- ½ cup crumbled feta cheese
- ¼ cup chopped red onion
- ¼ cup chopped Kalamata olives
- 2 tablespoons chopped fresh parsley
- 2 tablespoons extra-virgin olive oil
- 2 tablespoons red wine vinegar
- Salt and pepper to taste

Instructions:

1. In a large bowl, combine chickpeas, cucumber, tomatoes, feta, red onion, olives, and parsley.
2. In a small bowl, whisk together olive oil, red wine vinegar, salt, and pepper.
3. Pour the dressing over the salad and toss to coat.
4. Serve chilled or at room temperature.

Nutritional Information (per serving): *Calories: 350, Protein: 15g, Fat: 18g, Fiber: 12g*

2. Lemony Quinoa Salad with Asparagus and Dill

Servings: *2* ***Prep time:*** *20 minutes*

Ingredients:

- 1 cup quinoa, cooked and cooled
- 1 bunch asparagus, trimmed and cut into 1-inch pieces
- ½ cup chopped fresh dill
- ¼ cup chopped red onion
- ¼ cup toasted pine nuts
- 2 tablespoons extra-virgin olive oil
- 2 tablespoons lemon juice
- Salt and pepper to taste

Instructions:

1. Steam or roast asparagus until tender-crisp.
2. In a large bowl, combine quinoa, asparagus, dill, red onion, and pine nuts.
3. In a small bowl, whisk together olive oil, lemon juice, salt, and pepper.
4. Pour the dressing over the salad and toss to coat.
5. Serve chilled or at room temperature.

Nutritional Information *(per serving): Calories: 320, Protein: 10g, Fat: 15g, Fiber: 8g*

3. Kale Salad with Roasted Sweet Potato, Cranberries, and Pecans

Servings: *2* ***Prep time:*** *25 minutes*

Ingredients:

- 4 cups chopped kale
- 1 medium sweet potato, peeled and diced
- ½ cup dried cranberries
- ¼ cup chopped pecans
- 2 tablespoons extra-virgin olive oil
- 2 tablespoons balsamic vinegar
- 1 teaspoon Dijon mustard
- Salt and pepper to taste

Instructions:

1. Preheat oven to 400°F (200°C).
2. Toss sweet potato with 1 tablespoon olive oil, salt, and pepper. Spread on a baking sheet and roast for 20-25 minutes, or until tender.
3. In a large bowl, massage kale with remaining olive oil until softened.
4. Add roasted sweet potato, cranberries, pecans, balsamic vinegar, and Dijon mustard to the kale.
5. Toss to combine and season with salt and pepper to taste.

Nutritional Information (per serving): *Calories: 380, Protein: 8g, Fat: 20g, Fiber: 12g*

4. Black Bean and Corn Salad with Avocado Dressing

Servings: 2 **Prep time:** 15 minutes

Ingredients:

- 1 can (15 ounces) black beans, rinsed and drained
- 1 cup frozen or fresh corn kernels
- ½ cup chopped red onion
- ½ cup chopped red bell pepper
- ¼ cup chopped fresh cilantro
- 1 avocado, pitted and mashed
- 2 tablespoons lime juice
- Salt and pepper to taste

Instructions:

1. In a large bowl, combine black beans, corn, red onion, bell pepper, and cilantro.
2. In a small bowl, mash avocado with lime juice, salt, and pepper.
3. Pour the avocado dressing over the salad and toss to coat.

Nutritional Information (per serving): Calories: 310, Protein: 12g, Fat: 14g, Fiber: 15g

5. Roasted Beetroot and Goat Cheese Salad with Walnuts

Servings: *2* ***Prep time:*** *30 minutes*

Ingredients:

- 2 medium beetroots, scrubbed and trimmed
- 2 ounces goat cheese, crumbled
- ¼ cup chopped walnuts
- 2 cups mixed greens (arugula, spinach, or romaine lettuce)
- 2 tablespoons extra-virgin olive oil
- 1 tablespoon balsamic vinegar
- Salt and pepper to taste

Instructions:

1. Preheat oven to 400°F (200°C).
2. Wrap beetroots individually in aluminum foil and roast for 45-60 minutes, or until tender when pierced with a fork.
3. Let cool slightly, then peel and slice into wedges.
4. In a large bowl, combine mixed greens, beetroot, goat cheese, and walnuts.
5. Drizzle with olive oil and balsamic vinegar, and season with salt and pepper to taste.

Nutritional Information (per serving): *Calories: 360, Protein: 12g, Fat: 25g, Fiber: 8g*

6. Asian Slaw with Peanut Ginger Dressing

Servings: *4* ***Prep time:*** *20 minutes*

Ingredients:

- 1 small head of Napa cabbage, shredded
- 2 carrots, shredded
- 1 red bell pepper, thinly sliced
- ½ cup chopped fresh cilantro
- ¼ cup chopped peanuts
- ¼ cup rice vinegar
- 2 tablespoons soy sauce (or tamari for gluten-free)
- 1 tablespoon honey
- 1 tablespoon grated fresh ginger
- 1 clove garlic, minced
- 1 tablespoon sesame oil

Instructions:

1. In a large bowl, combine cabbage, carrots, bell pepper, and cilantro.
2. In a small bowl, whisk together rice vinegar, soy sauce, honey, ginger, garlic, and sesame oil.
3. Pour the dressing over the slaw and toss to coat.
4. Sprinkle with peanuts before serving.

Nutritional Information (per serving): *Calories: 200, Protein: 5g, Fat: 12g, Fiber: 5g*

7. White Bean and Spinach Salad with Lemon Vinaigrette

Servings: *2* ***Prep time:*** *15 minutes*

Ingredients:

- 1 can (15 ounces) cannellini beans, rinsed and drained
- 4 cups fresh baby spinach
- ½ cup cherry tomatoes, halved
- ¼ cup chopped red onion
- 2 tablespoons extra-virgin olive oil
- 2 tablespoons lemon juice
- 1 teaspoon Dijon mustard
- Salt and pepper to taste

Instructions:

1. In a large bowl, combine cannellini beans, spinach, tomatoes, and red onion.
2. In a small bowl, whisk together olive oil, lemon juice, Dijon mustard, salt, and pepper.
3. Pour the vinaigrette over the salad and toss to coat.

Nutritional Information (per serving): *Calories: 300, Protein: 12g, Fat: 15g, Fiber: 10g*

8. Tomato and Cucumber Salad with Fresh Basil

***Servings:** 2 **Prep time:** 10 minutes*

Ingredients:

- 2 tomatoes, chopped

- 1 cucumber, chopped

- ¼ cup chopped fresh basil

- 2 tablespoons extra-virgin olive oil

- 1 tablespoon red wine vinegar

- Salt and pepper to taste

Instructions:

1. Combine all ingredients in a bowl.

2. Toss to coat.

3. Serve chilled.

Nutritional Information (per serving): *Calories: 150, Protein: 2g, Fat: 12g, Fiber: 3g*

9. Roasted Brussels Sprouts with Balsamic Glaze

Servings: *2* ***Prep time:*** *25 minutes*

Ingredients:

- 1-pound Brussels sprouts, trimmed and halved
- 2 tablespoons olive oil
- Salt and pepper to taste
- 2 tablespoons balsamic vinegar
- 1 teaspoon honey

Instructions:

1. Preheat oven to 400°F (200°C).
2. Toss Brussels sprouts with olive oil, salt, and pepper.
3. Spread on a baking sheet and roast for 20-25 minutes, or until tender and browned.
4. In a small saucepan, heat balsamic vinegar and honey over medium heat until thickened.
5. Drizzle glaze over roasted Brussels sprouts and serve.

Nutritional Information (per serving): *Calories: 180, Protein: 5g, Fat: 12g, Fiber: 8g*

10. Roasted Carrots with Honey and Thyme

Servings: *2* ***Prep time:*** *30 minutes*

Ingredients:

- 1-pound carrots, peeled and cut into 1-inch pieces

- 2 tablespoons olive oil

- 1 tablespoon honey

- 1 teaspoon fresh thyme leaves

- Salt and pepper to taste

Instructions:

1. Preheat oven to 400°F (200°C).

2. Toss carrots with olive oil, honey, thyme, salt, and pepper.

3. Spread on a baking sheet and roast for 25-30 minutes, or until tender and caramelized.

Nutritional Information (per serving): *Calories: 160, Protein: 2g, Fat: 9g, Fiber: 5g*

11. Roasted Cauliflower and Chickpea Salad with Tahini Dressing

Servings: *2* ***Prep time:*** *35 minutes*

Ingredients:

- 1 head cauliflower, cut into florets
- 1 can (15 ounces) chickpeas, rinsed and drained
- 1 red onion, thinly sliced
- ¼ cup chopped fresh mint
- 2 tablespoons extra-virgin olive oil
- Salt and pepper to taste
- **Tahini Dressing:**
- ¼ cup tahini
- 2 tablespoons lemon juice
- 2 tablespoons water
- 1 clove garlic, minced
- Salt and pepper to taste

Instructions:

1. Preheat oven to 400°F (200°C).
2. Toss cauliflower florets with olive oil, salt, and pepper. Spread on a baking sheet and roast for 20-25 minutes, or until tender and slightly browned.
3. While cauliflower is roasting, whisk together tahini dressing ingredients in a small bowl.
4. In a large bowl, combine roasted cauliflower, chickpeas, red onion, and mint.

5. Drizzle with tahini dressing and toss to coat.

Nutritional Information (per serving): *Calories: 380, Protein: 14g, Fat: 22g, Fiber: 12g*

12. Mediterranean Lentil Salad with Cucumber, Tomatoes, and Herbs

Servings: *4* **Prep time:** *20 minutes*

Ingredients:

- 1 cup cooked brown lentils
- 1 cucumber, diced
- 1-pint cherry tomatoes, halved
- ¼ cup chopped red onion
- ½ cup chopped fresh parsley
- ¼ cup chopped fresh mint
- 2 tablespoons extra-virgin olive oil
- 2 tablespoons red wine vinegar
- Salt and pepper to taste

Instructions:

1. In a large bowl, combine lentils, cucumber, tomatoes, red onion, parsley, and mint.
2. In a small bowl, whisk together olive oil, red wine vinegar, salt, and pepper.
3. Pour dressing over salad and toss to coat.
4. Serve chilled or at room temperature.

Nutritional Information (per serving): *Calories: 210, Protein: 8g, Fat: 8g, Fiber: 9g*

13. Grilled Zucchini and Summer Squash with Pesto

Servings: *2* **Prep time:** *15 minutes*

Ingredients:

- 2 zucchinis, sliced lengthwise

- 2 yellow squash, sliced lengthwise

- 2 tablespoons olive oil

- Salt and pepper to taste

- ¼ cup prepared pesto

Instructions:

1. Preheat grill to medium heat.

2. Brush zucchini and squash slices with olive oil and season with salt and pepper.

3. Grill for 2-3 minutes per side, or until tender and slightly charred.

4. Serve with a dollop of pesto.

Nutritional Information (per serving): *Calories: 180, Protein: 3g, Fat: 15g, Fiber: 4g*

14. Roasted Asparagus with Lemon and Parmesan

Servings: *2* ***Prep time:*** *20 minutes*

Ingredients:

- 1 bunch asparagus, trimmed

- 1 tablespoon olive oil

- Salt and pepper to taste

- 1 lemon, zested and juiced

- 2 tablespoons grated Parmesan cheese

Instructions:

1. Preheat oven to 400°F (200°C).

2. Toss asparagus with olive oil, salt, and pepper.

3. Spread on a baking sheet and roast for 10-15 minutes, or until tender-crisp.

4. Drizzle with lemon juice and sprinkle with lemon zest and Parmesan cheese.

Nutritional Information (per serving): *Calories: 120, Protein: 5g, Fat: 8g, Fiber: 3g*

15. Roasted Sweet Potato Wedges with Spicy Yogurt Dip

Servings: *2* ***Prep time:*** *40 minutes*

Ingredients:

- 2 sweet potatoes, peeled and cut into wedges
- 2 tablespoons olive oil
- 1 teaspoon smoked paprika
- ½ teaspoon cumin
- Salt and pepper to taste
- ½ cup plain Greek yogurt
- 1 tablespoon chopped fresh cilantro
- ½ teaspoon sriracha (or other hot sauce)

Instructions:

1. Preheat oven to 400°F (200°C).
2. Toss sweet potato wedges with olive oil, paprika, cumin, salt, and pepper.
3. Spread on a baking sheet and roast for 25-30 minutes, or until tender and caramelized.
4. While sweet potatoes are roasting, combine yogurt, cilantro, and sriracha in a small bowl.
5. Serve sweet potato wedges with spicy yogurt dip.

Nutritional Information (per serving): *Calories: 280, Protein: 8g, Fat: 12g, Fiber: 7g*

16. Tomato and White Bean Soup with Kale and Rosemary

Servings: *2* ***Prep time:*** *30 minutes*

Ingredients:

- 1 tablespoon olive oil
- 1 onion, chopped
- 2 cloves garlic, minced
- 1 can (14 ounces) diced tomatoes, undrained
- 1 can (15 ounces) cannellini beans, rinsed and drained
- 4 cups vegetable broth
- 2 cups chopped kale
- 1 teaspoon dried rosemary
- Salt and pepper to taste

Instructions:

1. Heat olive oil in a large pot over medium heat.
2. Add onion and garlic and cook until softened, about 5 minutes.
3. Add tomatoes, beans, broth, kale, and rosemary.
4. Bring to a boil, then reduce heat and simmer for 15 minutes, or until kale is tender.
5. Season with salt and pepper to taste.

Nutritional Information (per serving): *Calories: 300, Protein: 15g, Fat: 8g, Fiber: 16g*

17. Hearty Vegetable and Barley Soup

Servings: *4* ***Prep time:*** *15 minutes* ***Cook time:*** *45 minutes*

Ingredients:

- 1 tablespoon olive oil
- 1 onion, chopped
- 2 carrots, chopped
- 2 stalks celery, chopped
- 2 cloves garlic, minced
- 6 cups vegetable broth
- ½ cup pearl barley
- 1 can (14.5 ounces) diced tomatoes, undrained
- 1 cup chopped kale
- ½ teaspoon dried thyme
- Salt and pepper to taste

Instructions:

1. Heat olive oil in a large pot over medium heat. Add onion, carrots, and celery and cook until softened, about 5 minutes.
2. Add garlic and cook for 1 minute more.
3. Stir in broth, barley, tomatoes, and thyme. Bring to a boil, then reduce heat and simmer for 30 minutes, or until barley is tender.
4. Stir in kale and cook for 5 minutes more, or until wilted.
5. Season with salt and pepper to taste.

Nutritional Information (per serving): *Calories: 250, Protein: 8g, Fat: 6g, Fiber: 12g*

18. Roasted Broccoli with Lemon and Garlic

Servings: *2* ***Prep time:*** *10 minutes* ***Cook time:*** *20 minutes*

- 1 head broccoli, cut into florets
- 2 tablespoons olive oil
- 2 cloves garlic, minced
- 1 lemon, zested and juiced
- Salt and pepper to taste

1. Preheat oven to 400°F (200°C).
2. Toss broccoli florets with olive oil, garlic, lemon zest, salt, and pepper.
3. Spread on a baking sheet and roast for 15-20 minutes, or until tender and slightly browned.
4. Drizzle with lemon juice before serving.

Nutritional Information (per serving): *Calories: 140, Protein: 4g, Fat: 10g, Fiber: 5g*

19. Greek Salad with Olives and Feta

Servings: *2* **Prep time:** *10 minutes*

Ingredients:

- 4 cups chopped romaine lettuce
- 1 cucumber, chopped
- 1 cup cherry tomatoes, halved
- ½ cup crumbled feta cheese
- ¼ cup chopped Kalamata olives
- ¼ cup chopped red onion
- 2 tablespoons extra-virgin olive oil
- 1 tablespoon red wine vinegar
- Dried oregano to taste
- Salt and pepper to taste

Instructions:

1. Combine all ingredients in a large bowl.

2. Toss to coat.

Nutritional Information (per serving): *Calories: 250, Protein: 10g, Fat: 18g, Fiber: 5g*

20. Caprese Salad with Balsamic Drizzle

Servings: *2* **Prep time:** *10 minutes*

Ingredients:

- 2 large tomatoes, sliced

- 8 ounces fresh mozzarella cheese, sliced

- 10 fresh basil leaves

- 2 tablespoons extra-virgin olive oil

- 1 tablespoon balsamic glaze

- Salt and pepper to taste

Instructions:

1. Arrange tomato and mozzarella slices on a platter, alternating between the two.

2. Top with basil leaves.

3. Drizzle with olive oil and balsamic glaze.

4. Season with salt and pepper to taste.

Nutritional Information (per serving): *Calories: 300, Protein: 15g, Fat: 22g, Fiber: 3g*

With this collection of 20 vibrant and flavorful salad, soup, and side dish recipes, you're well-equipped to embark on a culinary adventure that celebrates the MIND diet's principles. These dishes not only provide essential nutrients and antioxidants but also offer a symphony of tastes and textures to enliven your meals.

Chapter 4: Vegan and Vegetable Mains

"The earth has music for those who listen." This quote by George Santayana beautifully captures the essence of plant-based cuisine, where the symphony of flavors, colors, and textures harmonizes to create nourishing and delicious meals. In this chapter, we invite you to tune into the vibrant world of vegan and vegetable mains, where creativity and wellness intertwine.

The MIND diet embraces a plant-forward approach, recognizing the myriad benefits of vegetables, fruits, whole grains, and legumes for our brains and bodies. By incorporating these nutrient-dense foods into our main courses, we not only promote optimal health but also indulge in a culinary adventure that tantalizes the senses.

Let's embark on a journey through 20 unique vegan and vegetable main dish recipes that celebrate the MIND diet's principles of wholesome ingredients, diverse flavors, and effortless preparation. Whether you're a seasoned vegan, a curious vegetarian, or simply seeking to expand your culinary repertoire, you'll find an abundance of options to inspire and delight.

1. Moroccan Chickpea and Sweet Potato Stew

Servings: *2* ***Prep time:*** *15 minutes* ***Cook time:*** *30 minutes*

Ingredients:

- 1 tablespoon olive oil
- 1 onion, chopped
- 2 cloves garlic, minced
- 1 teaspoon ground cumin
- 1 teaspoon ground coriander
- ½ teaspoon turmeric
- ¼ teaspoon cayenne pepper
- 1 sweet potato, peeled and diced
- 1 can (14.5 ounces) diced tomatoes, undrained
- 1 can (15 ounces) chickpeas, rinsed and drained
- 1 cup vegetable broth
- ½ cup chopped fresh cilantro
- Salt and pepper to taste

Instructions:

1. Heat olive oil in a large pot over medium heat. Add onion and cook until softened, about 5 minutes.
2. Add garlic, cumin, coriander, turmeric, and cayenne pepper and cook for 1 minute more.

3. Stir in sweet potato, tomatoes, chickpeas, and broth. Bring to a boil, then reduce heat and simmer for 20 minutes, or until sweet potatoes are tender.
4. Stir in cilantro and season with salt and pepper to taste.

Nutritional Information (per serving): *Calories: 450, Protein: 15g, Fat: 12g, Fiber: 18g*

2. Mediterranean Stuffed Eggplant

***Servings:** 2 **Prep time:** 20 minutes **Cook time:** 45 minutes*

Ingredients:

- 2 small eggplants, halved lengthwise
- 1 tablespoon olive oil
- 1 onion, chopped
- 2 cloves garlic, minced
- 1 cup chopped mushrooms
- ½ cup cooked brown rice
- ½ cup chopped tomatoes
- ¼ cup chopped fresh parsley
- ¼ cup crumbled feta cheese
- Salt and pepper to taste

Instructions:

1. Preheat oven to 375°F (190°C).
2. Scoop out the flesh of the eggplants, leaving a ½-inch border. Chop the eggplant flesh and set aside.
3. Brush eggplant halves with olive oil and season with salt and pepper. Place cut-side down on a baking sheet and bake for 20 minutes.
4. While eggplants are baking, heat olive oil in a pan over medium heat. Add onion and cook until softened, about 5 minutes.
5. Add garlic and mushrooms and cook until softened, about 5 minutes more.

6. Stir in chopped eggplant flesh, rice, tomatoes, parsley, and feta cheese. Season with salt and pepper to taste.
7. Fill eggplant halves with the stuffing and bake for 25 minutes more, or until eggplant is tender and stuffing is heated through.

Nutritional Information (per serving): *Calories: 350, Protein: 12g, Fat: 18g, Fiber: 10g*

3. Lentil and Vegetable Curry

Servings: *4* ***Prep time:*** *15 minutes* ***Cook time:*** *30 minutes*

Ingredients:

- 1 tablespoon olive oil
- 1 onion, chopped
- 2 cloves garlic, minced
- 1 tablespoon curry powder
- ½ teaspoon ground ginger
- ¼ teaspoon cayenne pepper (optional)
- 1 sweet potato, peeled and diced
- 1 red bell pepper, diced
- 1 can (14.5 ounces) diced tomatoes, undrained
- 1 cup red lentils
- 2 cups vegetable broth
- ½ cup chopped fresh cilantro
- Salt and pepper to taste

Instructions:

1. Heat olive oil in a large pot over medium heat. Add onion and cook until softened, about 5 minutes.
2. Add garlic, curry powder, ginger, and cayenne pepper (if using) and cook for 1 minute more.
3. Stir in sweet potato, bell pepper, tomatoes, lentils, and broth. Bring to a boil, then reduce heat and simmer for 20-25 minutes, or until lentils and vegetables are tender.

4. Stir in cilantro and season with salt and pepper
   to taste.

Nutritional Information (per serving): *Calories:
350, Protein: 15g, Fat: 8g, Fiber: 16g*

4. Vegetable Paella with Saffron and Artichoke Hearts

Servings: *4* ***Prep time:*** *20 minutes* ***Cook time:*** *45 minutes*

Ingredients:

- 1 tablespoon olive oil
- 1 onion, chopped
- 2 cloves garlic, minced
- 1 red bell pepper, diced
- 1 yellow bell pepper, diced
- 1 cup Arborio rice
- 2 ½ cups vegetable broth
- ½ teaspoon saffron threads
- 1 jar (14 ounces) artichoke hearts, drained and quartered
- ½ cup frozen peas
- ¼ cup chopped fresh parsley
- Salt and pepper to taste

Instructions:

1. Heat olive oil in a large skillet or paella pan over medium heat. Add onion and cook until softened, about 5 minutes.
2. Add garlic and bell peppers and cook until softened, about 5 minutes more.
3. Stir in rice and cook for 1 minute.

4. Add broth, saffron threads, artichoke hearts, peas, and parsley. Season with salt and pepper to taste.
5. Bring to a boil, then reduce heat and simmer for 20 minutes, or until rice is tender and liquid is absorbed.
6. Remove from heat and let stand for 5 minutes before serving.

Nutritional Information (per serving): *Calories: 380, Protein: 10g, Fat: 12g, Fiber: 10g*

5. Sweet Potato and Black Bean Burgers with Avocado Crema

Servings: 4 **Prep time:** *20 minutes* **Cook time:** *15 minutes*

Ingredients:

- 1 tablespoon olive oil
- 1 onion, chopped
- 2 cloves garlic, minced
- 1 teaspoon chili powder
- ½ teaspoon cumin
- ¼ teaspoon smoked paprika
- 1 sweet potato, peeled and grated
- 1 can (15 ounces) black beans, rinsed and drained
- ½ cup breadcrumbs
- ¼ cup chopped fresh cilantro
- Salt and pepper to taste
- **Avocado Crema:**
- 1 avocado, pitted and mashed
- 2 tablespoons lime juice
- 2 tablespoons plain Greek yogurt
- Salt and pepper to taste

Instructions:

1. Heat olive oil in a skillet over medium heat. Add onion and cook until softened, about 5 minutes.

2. Add garlic, chili powder, cumin, and smoked paprika and cook for 1 minute more.
3. In a large bowl, combine sweet potato, black beans, breadcrumbs, cilantro, and the cooked onion mixture. Season with salt and pepper to taste.
4. Form mixture into 4 patties.
5. Heat olive oil in a skillet over medium heat. Cook patties for 5-7 minutes per side, or until golden brown and cooked through.
6. While patties are cooking, prepare avocado crema by mashing avocado with lime juice, yogurt, salt, and pepper.
7. Serve burgers on whole-wheat buns or lettuce wraps with avocado crema.

Nutritional Information (per serving): *Calories: 400, Protein: 18g, Fat: 15g, Fiber: 12g*

6. Portobello Mushroom Fajitas

Servings: *2* ***Prep time:*** *15 minutes* ***Cook time:*** *20 minutes*

Ingredients:

- 2 large portobello mushrooms, stems removed and sliced
- 1 bell pepper (any color), sliced
- 1 onion, sliced
- 1 tablespoon olive oil
- 1 teaspoon chili powder
- ½ teaspoon cumin
- ¼ teaspoon smoked paprika
- Salt and pepper to taste
- Whole-wheat tortillas
- Optional toppings: avocado, salsa, guacamole, shredded lettuce, chopped tomatoes

Instructions:

1. Heat olive oil in a large skillet over medium heat.
2. Add mushrooms, bell pepper, and onion and cook, stirring occasionally, until softened and slightly browned, about 10 minutes.
3. Stir in chili powder, cumin, smoked paprika, salt, and pepper.

4. Warm tortillas in a dry skillet or microwave.

5. Fill tortillas with mushroom mixture and desired toppings.

Nutritional Information (per serving without toppings): *Calories: 280, Protein: 10g, Fat: 12g, Fiber: 8g*

7. Vegetable Stir-Fry with Tofu and Peanut Sauce

Servings: *2* ***Prep time:*** *15 minutes* ***Cook time:*** *20 minutes*

Ingredients:

- 1 block extra-firm tofu, pressed and cubed
- 1 tablespoon olive oil
- 1 onion, sliced
- 2 cloves garlic, minced
- 1 red bell pepper, sliced
- 1 head broccoli, cut into florets
- **Peanut Sauce:**
- ¼ cup peanut butter
- 2 tablespoons soy sauce (or tamari for gluten-free)
- 2 tablespoons water
- 1 tablespoon rice vinegar
- 1 teaspoon honey
- ½ teaspoon grated fresh ginger
- Pinch of red pepper flakes
- Cooked brown rice or noodles for serving (optional)

Instructions:

1. Heat olive oil in a large skillet or wok over medium heat.

2. Add tofu and cook, stirring occasionally, until golden brown on all sides, about 10 minutes.
3. Add onion, garlic, bell pepper, and broccoli and cook, stirring constantly, until vegetables are tender-crisp, about 5 minutes.
4. While vegetables are cooking, whisk together peanut sauce ingredients in a small bowl.
5. Pour peanut sauce over the stir-fry and cook for 1 minute more, or until heated through.
6. Serve over rice or noodles, if desired.

Nutritional Information (per serving without rice or noodles): *Calories: 450, Protein: 25g, Fat: 28g, Fiber: 10g*

8. Butternut Squash and Black Bean Enchiladas

Servings: *4* **Prep Time:** *25 minutes* **Cook Time:* *30 minutes*

Ingredients:

- 1 butternut squash, peeled, seeded, and cubed
- 1 tablespoon olive oil
- 1 onion, chopped
- 2 cloves garlic, minced
- 1 teaspoon chili powder
- ½ teaspoon cumin
- ¼ teaspoon smoked paprika
- 1 can (15 ounces) black beans, rinsed and drained
- ½ cup corn kernels (fresh or frozen)
- 8 whole-wheat tortillas
- 1 cup enchilada sauce
- ½ cup shredded Monterey Jack cheese (optional)

Instructions:

1. Preheat oven to 375°F (190°C).

2. Toss butternut squash with olive oil, salt, and pepper. Spread on a baking sheet and roast for 20-25 minutes, or until tender.

3. While squash is roasting, heat olive oil in a skillet over medium heat. Add onion and cook until softened, about 5 minutes.

4. Add garlic, chili powder, cumin, and paprika and cook for 1 minute more.

5. Stir in black beans and corn and cook until heated through.

6. Mash roasted butternut squash with a fork.

7. Spread a thin layer of enchilada sauce on the bottom of a baking dish.

8. Fill each tortilla with a spoonful of mashed squash and black bean mixture. Roll up and place seam-side down in the baking dish.

9. Pour remaining enchilada sauce over the enchiladas and sprinkle with cheese, if using.

10. Bake for 15-20 minutes, or until heated through and cheese is melted.

Nutritional Information (per serving without cheese): *Calories: 420, Protein: 16g, Fat: 12g, Fiber: 15g*

9. Spicy Thai Red Curry with Tofu and Vegetables

Servings: *2* ***Prep time:*** *15 minutes* ***Cook time:*** *25 minutes*

Ingredients:

- 1 block extra-firm tofu, pressed and cubed
- 1 tablespoon olive oil
- 1 onion, sliced
- 2 cloves garlic, minced
- 1 tablespoon red curry paste
- 1 can (14 ounces) coconut milk
- ½ cup vegetable broth
- 1 red bell pepper, sliced
- 1 head broccoli, cut into florets
- ½ cup snow peas
- 1 tablespoon fish sauce (or soy sauce for vegan)
- 1 tablespoon lime juice
- Fresh basil leaves for garnish

Instructions:

1. Heat olive oil in a large skillet or wok over medium heat. Add tofu and cook, stirring occasionally, until golden brown on all sides, about 10 minutes.
2. Add onion and garlic and cook until softened, about 5 minutes.

3. Stir in red curry paste and cook for 1 minute more.
4. Add coconut milk, broth, bell pepper, broccoli, and snow peas. Bring to a boil, then reduce heat and simmer for 10 minutes, or until vegetables are tender.
5. Stir in fish sauce (or soy sauce) and lime juice.
6. Serve over cooked brown rice or quinoa, garnished with fresh basil.

Nutritional Information (per serving without rice or quinoa): *Calories: 480, Protein: 20g, Fat: 35g, Fiber: 12g*

10. Spinach and Artichoke Stuffed Shells

Servings: *4* ***Prep time:*** *20 minutes* ***Cook time:*** *35 minutes*

Ingredients:

- 1 box (12 ounces) jumbo pasta shells
- 1 jar (14 ounces) artichoke hearts, drained and chopped
- 1 package (10 ounces) frozen chopped spinach, thawed and squeezed dry
- 1 container (15 ounces) ricotta cheese
- ½ cup grated Parmesan cheese
- 2 cloves garlic, minced
- 1 teaspoon dried oregano
- Salt and pepper to taste
- 1 jar (24 ounces) marinara sauce

Instructions:

1. Preheat oven to 375°F (190°C).
2. Cook pasta shells according to package directions. Drain and rinse with cold water.
3. In a large bowl, combine artichoke hearts, spinach, ricotta, Parmesan, garlic, oregano, salt, and pepper.

4. Spread a thin layer of marinara sauce on the bottom of a baking dish.
5. Fill each pasta shell with the spinach and artichoke mixture. Arrange stuffed shells in the baking dish.
6. Pour remaining marinara sauce over the shells.
7. Bake for 25-30 minutes, or until heated through and bubbly.

Nutritional Information (per serving): *Calories: 400, Protein: 18g, Fat: 15g, Fiber: 8g*

11. Vegan Shepherd's Pie with Lentils and Mushrooms

Servings: *4* ***Prep time:*** *20 minutes* ***Cook time:*** *45 minutes*

Ingredients:

- 1 tablespoon olive oil
- 1 onion, chopped
- 2 cloves garlic, minced
- 8 ounces mushrooms, sliced
- 1 cup green lentils
- 2 cups vegetable broth
- 1 tablespoon tomato paste
- 1 teaspoon dried thyme
- 1 teaspoon dried rosemary
- Salt and pepper to taste
- **Mashed Potato Topping:**
- 2 pounds russet potatoes, peeled and cut into chunks
- ½ cup unsweetened almond milk
- 2 tablespoons vegan butter
- Salt and pepper to taste

Instructions:

1. Preheat oven to 375°F (190°C).
2. Heat olive oil in a large skillet over medium heat. Add onion and cook until softened, about 5 minutes.
3. Add garlic and mushrooms and cook until softened, about 5 minutes more.
4. Stir in lentils, broth, tomato paste, thyme, rosemary, salt, and pepper. Bring to a boil, then reduce heat and simmer for 20 minutes, or until lentils are tender.
5. While lentils are cooking, prepare mashed potato topping. Boil potatoes until tender. Drain and

mash with almond milk and vegan butter. Season with salt and pepper to taste.

6. Spread lentil mixture in a baking dish. Top with mashed potatoes.
7. Bake for 20-25 minutes, or until heated through and potatoes are golden brown.

Nutritional Information (per serving): *Calories: 450, Protein: 18g, Fat: 12g, Fiber: 15g*

12. Summer Vegetable Tian

Servings: *4* ***Prep time:*** *20 minutes* ***Cook time:*** *45 minutes*

Ingredients:

- 2 zucchinis, thinly sliced
- 2 yellow squash, thinly sliced
- 2 tomatoes, thinly sliced
- 1 red onion, thinly sliced
- 2 cloves garlic, minced
- 2 tablespoons olive oil
- 1 teaspoon dried oregano
- 1 teaspoon dried basil
- Salt and pepper to taste
- ¼ cup grated Parmesan cheese (optional)

Instructions:

1. Preheat oven to 375°F (190°C).
2. Arrange zucchini, squash, tomatoes, and onion in overlapping slices in a round baking dish.
3. Sprinkle with garlic, oregano, basil, salt, and pepper.
4. Drizzle with olive oil.
5. Bake for 45 minutes, or until vegetables are tender and lightly browned.

6. Sprinkle with Parmesan cheese, if using, before
    serving.

**Nutritional Information (per serving without
cheese):** *Calories: 150, Protein: 4g, Fat: 9g, Fiber:
5g*

13. Spicy Black Bean and Avocado Tacos

Servings: *2* ***Prep time:*** *15 minutes*

Ingredients:

- 1 tablespoon olive oil
- 1 onion, chopped
- 2 cloves garlic, minced
- 1 teaspoon chili powder
- ½ teaspoon cumin
- ¼ teaspoon smoked paprika
- 1 can (15 ounces) black beans, rinsed and drained
- ½ cup salsa
- 1 avocado, sliced
- 4 corn tortillas, warmed
- Optional toppings: shredded lettuce, chopped tomatoes, chopped cilantro, hot sauce

Instructions:

1. Heat olive oil in a skillet over medium heat. Add onion and cook until softened, about 5 minutes.
2. Add garlic, chili powder, cumin, and paprika and cook for 1 minute more.
3. Stir in black beans and salsa. Heat through.

4. Fill tortillas with black bean mixture, avocado slices, and desired toppings.

Nutritional Information (per serving without toppings): *Calories: 350, Protein: 12g, Fat: 15g, Fiber: 12g*

14. Quinoa-Stuffed Bell Peppers

***Servings:** 2 **Prep time:** 15 minutes **Cook time:** 40 minutes*

Ingredients:

- 2 bell peppers (any color)
- 1 cup cooked quinoa
- ½ cup chopped mushrooms
- ½ cup chopped zucchini
- ¼ cup chopped onion
- 1 tablespoon olive oil
- ½ teaspoon dried oregano
- ½ teaspoon dried basil
- Salt and pepper to taste
- ¼ cup shredded vegan cheese (optional)

Instructions:

1. Preheat oven to 375°F (190°C).
2. Cut bell peppers in half lengthwise and remove seeds and membranes.
3. Heat olive oil in a skillet over medium heat. Add onion and cook until softened, about 5 minutes.
4. Add mushrooms and zucchini and cook until softened, about 5 minutes more.
5. Stir in quinoa, oregano, basil, salt, and pepper.

6. Fill bell pepper halves with quinoa mixture.

7. Place in a baking dish and bake for 30-35 minutes, or until peppers are tender.

8. Top with vegan cheese, if using, and bake for 5 minutes more, or until cheese is melted.

Nutritional Information (per serving without cheese): *Calories: 300, Protein: 10g, Fat: 12g, Fiber: 10g*

15. Spicy Peanut Noodles with Vegetables

Servings: *2* ***Prep time:*** *10 minutes* ***Cook time:*** *15 minutes*

Ingredients:

- 8 ounces whole-wheat spaghetti
- 1 tablespoon olive oil
- 1 red bell pepper, thinly sliced
- ½ cup snow peas
- ¼ cup chopped peanuts
- **Peanut Sauce:**
- ¼ cup peanut butter
- 2 tablespoons soy sauce (or tamari for gluten-free)
- 2 tablespoons water
- 1 tablespoon rice vinegar
- 1 teaspoon honey
- ½ teaspoon grated fresh ginger
- Pinch of red pepper flakes

Instructions:

1. Cook spaghetti according to package directions. Drain and rinse with cold water.
2. While spaghetti is cooking, heat olive oil in a large skillet or wok over medium heat.

3. Add bell pepper and snow peas and cook, stirring constantly, until tender-crisp, about 5 minutes.

4. In a small bowl, whisk together peanut sauce ingredients.

5. Add spaghetti, peanut sauce, and peanuts to the skillet with vegetables. Toss to coat.

6. Serve warm.

Nutritional Information (per serving): *Calories: 550, Protein: 20g, Fat: 25g, Fiber: 12g*

16. Spicy Tofu Scramble with Black Beans and Sweet Potatoes

*Servings: 2 **Prep time:** 10 minutes **Cook time:** 20 minutes*

Ingredients:

- 1 tablespoon olive oil

- 1 onion, chopped

- 2 cloves garlic, minced

- 1 teaspoon chili powder

- ½ teaspoon cumin

- ¼ teaspoon smoked paprika

- 1 sweet potato, peeled and diced

- 1 block extra-firm tofu, crumbled

- 1 can (15 ounces) black beans, rinsed and drained

- ½ cup salsa

- ¼ cup chopped fresh cilantro

- Salt and pepper to taste

- Optional toppings: avocado slices, hot sauce, shredded vegan cheese

Instructions:

1. Heat olive oil in a large skillet over medium heat. Add onion and cook until softened, about 5 minutes.

2. Add garlic, chili powder, cumin, and paprika and cook for 1 minute more.

3. Stir in sweet potato and cook for 5-7 minutes, or until tender.

4. Add tofu and black beans and cook until heated through.

5. Stir in salsa and cilantro. Season with salt and pepper to taste.

6. Serve warm with desired toppings.

Nutritional Information (per serving without toppings): *Calories: 400, Protein: 20g, Fat: 18g, Fiber: 15g*

17. Vegan Stuffed Grape Leaves (Dolmas)

Servings: *4* **Prep time:** *30 minutes* **Cook time:** *45 minutes*

Ingredients:

- 1 jar (16 ounces) grape leaves, rinsed
- 1 cup cooked brown rice
- ½ cup chopped fresh herbs (parsley, dill, mint)
- ¼ cup chopped red onion
- ¼ cup chopped tomatoes
- 2 tablespoons lemon juice
- 2 tablespoons olive oil
- Salt and pepper to taste

Instructions:

1. In a large bowl, combine rice, herbs, onion, tomatoes, lemon juice, olive oil, salt, and pepper.

2. Lay a grape leaf flat on a work surface, vein side up. Place a tablespoon of filling in the center of the leaf.

3. Fold the bottom of the leaf over the filling, then fold in the sides. Roll up tightly.

4. Repeat with remaining grape leaves and filling.

5. Place stuffed grape leaves in a single layer in a pot. Add enough water to cover them by 1 inch.

6. Bring to a boil, then reduce heat and simmer for 45 minutes, or until grape leaves are tender.

7. Serve warm or cold.

Nutritional Information (per serving): *Calories: 150, Protein: 4g, Fat: 6g, Fiber: 5g*

18. Cauliflower Steaks with Lemon Herb Sauce

***Servings:** 2 **Prep time:** 10 minutes **Cook time:** 25 minutes*

Ingredients:

- 1 head cauliflower, cut into 1-inch thick "steaks"
- 2 tablespoons olive oil
- Salt and pepper to taste
- **Lemon Herb Sauce:**
- ¼ cup chopped fresh parsley
- ¼ cup chopped fresh dill
- 2 tablespoons lemon juice
- 2 tablespoons olive oil
- 1 clove garlic, minced
- Salt and pepper to taste

Instructions:

1. Preheat oven to 400°F (200°C).
2. Brush cauliflower steaks with olive oil and season with salt and pepper.
3. Place on a baking sheet and roast for 15-20 minutes per side, or until tender and lightly browned.

4. While cauliflower is roasting, whisk together lemon herb sauce ingredients in a small bowl.

5. Serve cauliflower steaks with lemon herb sauce drizzled on top.

Nutritional Information (per serving): *Calories: 250, Protein: 6g, Fat: 18g, Fiber: 7g*

19. Sweet Potato and Chickpea Buddha Bowl

***Servings:** 2 **Prep time:** 20 minutes*

Ingredients:

- 1 sweet potato, peeled and cubed
- 1 tablespoon olive oil
- ½ teaspoon cumin
- ½ teaspoon paprika
- Salt and pepper to taste
- 1 can (15 ounces) chickpeas, rinsed and drained
- 1 cup chopped kale
- ½ avocado, sliced
- ¼ cup chopped red onion
- ¼ cup crumbled feta cheese
- 2 tablespoons tahini dressing

Instructions:

1. Preheat oven to 400°F (200°C).
2. Toss sweet potato cubes with olive oil, cumin, paprika, salt, and pepper. Spread on a baking sheet and roast for 20-25 minutes, or until tender and slightly browned.
3. While sweet potatoes are roasting, massage kale with a drizzle of olive oil and a pinch of salt.

4. To assemble bowls, divide quinoa, roasted sweet
   potatoes, chickpeas, kale, avocado slices, red
   onion, and feta cheese among two bowls. Drizzle
   with tahini dressing.

Nutritional Information (per serving): *Calories:
480, Protein: 16g, Fat: 25g, Fiber: 15g*

20. Lentil Sloppy Joes

Servings: *4* ***Prep time:*** *15 minutes* ***Cook time:*** *25 minutes*

Ingredients:

- 1 tablespoon olive oil
- 1 onion, chopped
- 2 cloves garlic, minced
- 1 green bell pepper, chopped
- 1 teaspoon chili powder
- ½ teaspoon cumin
- ¼ teaspoon smoked paprika
- 1 cup cooked brown lentils
- 1 can (14.5 ounces) diced tomatoes, undrained
- ½ cup ketchup
- 2 tablespoons brown sugar
- 1 tablespoon apple cider vinegar
- Salt and pepper to taste
- Whole-wheat hamburger buns

Instructions:

1. Heat olive oil in a large skillet over medium heat. Add onion and cook until softened, about 5 minutes.

2. Add garlic, bell pepper, chili powder, cumin, and paprika and cook for 1 minute more.

3. Stir in lentils, tomatoes, ketchup, brown sugar, and vinegar. Bring to a boil, then reduce heat and simmer for 15 minutes, or until thickened. Season with salt and pepper to taste.

4. Serve on whole-wheat hamburger buns.

Nutritional Information (per serving without bun): Calories: 300, Protein: 14g, Fat: 5g, Fiber: 15g

Embrace the vibrant flavors, diverse textures, and wholesome ingredients of these 20 vegan and vegetable mains, and discover a world of culinary possibilities that nourish your body and delight your taste buds.

Chapter 5: Fish and Seafood Mains

"There is no sincerer love than the love of food." George Bernard Shaw's declaration rings true for many, and the MIND diet embraces this love, especially when it comes to fish and seafood. These treasures from the sea offer a bounty of flavors, textures, and nutrients that are vital for brain health and overall well-being.

As we delve into this chapter, we'll cast our nets wide, exploring a diverse array of fish and seafood main dishes that celebrate the MIND diet's principles. You'll find recipes that span various culinary traditions, each one showcasing the unique characteristics of different types of fish and shellfish. From flaky white fish to succulent salmon, from delicate scallops to hearty shrimp, there's a dish to entice every palate and elevate your dining experience.

Get ready to embark on a culinary adventure that takes you from the shores of the Mediterranean to the coasts of Asia, all while staying true to the MIND diet's emphasis on wholesome ingredients and simple preparation. Let's dive in and discover 20 unique fish and seafood mains that will nourish your body and delight your senses.

1. Lemon Herb Baked Salmon

Servings: *2* ***Prep time:*** *10 minutes* ***Cook time:*** *20 minutes*

Ingredients:

- 2 (6-ounce) salmon fillets
- 2 tablespoons olive oil
- 2 tablespoons lemon juice
- 2 cloves garlic, minced
- 1 tablespoon chopped fresh dill
- 1 tablespoon chopped fresh parsley
- Salt and pepper to taste

Instructions:

1. Preheat oven to 400°F (200°C).
2. Place salmon fillets on a baking sheet lined with parchment paper.
3. In a small bowl, whisk together olive oil, lemon juice, garlic, dill, parsley, salt, and pepper.
4. Drizzle the mixture over the salmon fillets.
5. Bake for 15-20 minutes, or until the salmon is cooked through and flakes easily with a fork.

Nutritional Information (per serving): *Calories: 350, Protein: 30g, Fat: 20g*

2. Mediterranean Baked Cod with Tomatoes, Olives, and Capers

Servings: *2* ***Prep time:*** *15 minutes* ***Cook time:*** *25 minutes*

Ingredients:

- 2 (6-ounce) cod fillets
- 1 tablespoon olive oil
- 1 cup chopped tomatoes
- ¼ cup chopped Kalamata olives
- 1 tablespoon capers
- 2 cloves garlic, minced
- ½ teaspoon dried oregano
- Salt and pepper to taste

Instructions:

1. Preheat oven to 400°F (200°C).
2. Place cod fillets on a baking sheet lined with parchment paper.
3. In a bowl, combine tomatoes, olives, capers, garlic, oregano, salt, and pepper.
4. Spoon the tomato mixture over the cod fillets.
5. Drizzle with olive oil.
6. Bake for 20-25 minutes, or until the fish is cooked through and flakes easily with a fork.

Nutritional Information (per serving): *Calories: 280, Protein: 25g, Fat: 12g*

3. Garlic Butter Shrimp Scampi with Zucchini Noodles

Servings: *2* **Prep time:** *15 minutes* **Cook time:** *15 minutes*

Ingredients:

- 1-pound large shrimp, peeled and deveined
- 2 tablespoons olive oil
- 4 cloves garlic, minced
- ½ cup dry white wine
- 2 tablespoons lemon juice
- 2 tablespoons chopped fresh parsley
- Salt and pepper to taste
- 2 medium zucchinis, spiralized into noodles

Instructions:

1. Heat olive oil in a large skillet over medium heat. Add shrimp and cook until pink and opaque, about 3-4 minutes per side. Remove shrimp from skillet and set aside.

2. Add garlic to the skillet and cook for 30 seconds, or until fragrant.

3. Stir in white wine and lemon juice. Bring to a simmer and cook for 2 minutes, or until slightly reduced.

4. Add zucchini noodles to the skillet and cook for 2-3 minutes, or until tender-crisp.
5. Return shrimp to the skillet and stir in parsley, salt, and pepper.
6. Serve immediately.

Nutritional Information (per serving): *Calories: 350, Protein: 35g, Fat: 15g*

4. Spicy Tuna Salad with Avocado and Lime

Servings: *2* ***Prep time:*** *10 minutes*

Ingredients:

- 2 cans (5 ounces) tuna in water, drained
- ½ avocado, diced
- ½ cup chopped celery
- ¼ cup chopped red onion
- 2 tablespoons chopped fresh cilantro
- 2 tablespoons lime juice
- 1 tablespoon mayonnaise (optional)
- ½ teaspoon sriracha (or other hot sauce, adjust to taste)
- Salt and pepper to taste

Instructions:

1. In a medium bowl, combine tuna, avocado, celery, red onion, and cilantro.
2. In a small bowl, whisk together lime juice, mayonnaise (if using), sriracha, salt, and pepper.
3. Pour the dressing over the tuna mixture and stir to combine.
4. Serve on whole-wheat bread, lettuce cups, or crackers.

Nutritional Information (per serving without bread): *Calories: 250, Protein: 25g, Fat: 12g*

5. Pan-Seared Scallops with Brown Butter and Sage

Servings: *2* ***Prep time:*** *5 minutes* ***Cook time:*** *10 minutes*

Ingredients:

- 1-pound sea scallops, patted dry
- 2 tablespoons olive oil
- 4 tablespoons butter
- 6-8 fresh sage leaves
- Salt and pepper to taste

Instructions:

1. Heat olive oil in a large skillet over medium-high heat.
2. Season scallops with salt and pepper.
3. Add scallops to the skillet and cook for 2-3 minutes per side, or until golden brown and opaque. Remove scallops from the skillet and set aside.
4. Add butter to the skillet and cook over medium heat until melted and browned.
5. Add sage leaves and cook for 1 minute, or until fragrant.
6. Return scallops to the skillet and toss to coat in the brown butter and sage.
7. Serve immediately.

Nutritional Information (per serving): *Calories: 380, Protein: 25g, Fat: 25g*

6. Blackened Tilapia with Mango Salsa

***Servings:** 2 **Prep time:** 15 minutes **Cook time:** 10 minutes*

Ingredients:

- 2 (6-ounce) tilapia fillets

- 1 tablespoon blackened seasoning

- 1 tablespoon olive oil

- **Mango Salsa:**

- 1 ripe mango, diced

- ½ cup chopped red onion

- ¼ cup chopped fresh cilantro

- 2 tablespoons lime juice

- ½ jalapeno, seeded and minced (optional)

- Salt and pepper to taste

Instructions:

1. Pat tilapia fillets dry and sprinkle with blackened seasoning.

2. Heat olive oil in a large skillet over medium-high heat.

3. Add tilapia fillets to the skillet and cook for 3-4 minutes per side, or until cooked through and flaky.

4. While fish is cooking, combine mango salsa ingredients in a bowl.

5. Serve tilapia topped with mango salsa.

Nutritional Information (per serving): *Calories: 300, Protein: 25g, Fat: 10g*

7. Salmon with Roasted Grapes and Balsamic Reduction

Servings: *2* ***Prep time:*** *10 minutes* ***Cook time:*** *25 minutes*

Ingredients:

- 2 (6-ounce) salmon fillets
- 1 cup red grapes
- 2 tablespoons olive oil
- 2 tablespoons balsamic vinegar
- 1 teaspoon Dijon mustard
- Salt and pepper to taste

Instructions:

1. Preheat oven to 400°F (200°C).
2. Place salmon fillets on a baking sheet lined with parchment paper.
3. In a bowl, toss grapes with 1 tablespoon olive oil, salt, and pepper. Spread around the salmon fillets.
4. Roast for 15-20 minutes, or until salmon is cooked through and grapes are softened.
5. While salmon and grapes are roasting, whisk together balsamic vinegar, Dijon mustard, and remaining olive oil in a small saucepan. Bring to

a simmer and cook for 5 minutes, or until thickened.

6. Drizzle balsamic reduction over salmon and grapes before serving.

Nutritional Information (per serving): *Calories: 400, Protein: 30g, Fat: 25g*

8. Mediterranean Tuna Salad with White Beans and Artichoke Hearts

Servings: 2 Prep time: 15 minutes

Ingredients:

- 2 cans (5 ounces) tuna in olive oil, drained
- 1 can (15 ounces) cannellini beans, rinsed and drained
- ½ cup chopped artichoke hearts
- ¼ cup chopped red onion
- ¼ cup chopped fresh parsley
- 2 tablespoons lemon juice
- 2 tablespoons olive oil
- Salt and pepper to taste

Instructions:

1. In a medium bowl, combine tuna, cannellini beans, artichoke hearts, red onion, and parsley.
2. In a small bowl, whisk together lemon juice, olive oil, salt, and pepper.
3. Pour the dressing over the tuna mixture and stir to combine.
4. Serve on whole-wheat bread, lettuce cups, or crackers.

Nutritional Information (per serving without bread): *Calories: 350, Protein: 28g, Fat: 18g*

9. Spicy Shrimp Tacos with Avocado Crema

Servings: *2* ***Prep time:*** *15 minutes* ***Cook time:*** *10 minutes*

Ingredients:

- 1-pound large shrimp, peeled and deveined
- 1 tablespoon olive oil
- 1 teaspoon chili powder
- ½ teaspoon cumin
- ¼ teaspoon smoked paprika
- Salt and pepper to taste
- 4 corn tortillas, warmed
- **Avocado Crema:**
- 1 avocado, pitted and mashed
- 2 tablespoons lime juice
- 2 tablespoons plain Greek yogurt
- Salt and pepper to taste
- Optional toppings: shredded cabbage, chopped tomatoes, chopped cilantro, hot sauce

Instructions:

1. Toss shrimp with olive oil, chili powder, cumin, paprika, salt, and pepper.

2. Heat a large skillet over medium-high heat. Add shrimp and cook for 2-3 minutes per side, or until pink and opaque.

3. While shrimp is cooking, prepare avocado crema by mashing avocado with lime juice, yogurt, salt, and pepper.

4. Fill tortillas with shrimp, avocado crema, and desired toppings.

Nutritional Information (per serving without toppings): *Calories: 380, Protein: 25g, Fat: 20g*

10. Baked Flounder with Lemon and Herbs

Servings: *2* **Prep time:** *10 minutes* **Cook time:** *20 minutes*

Ingredients:

- 2 (6-ounce) flounder fillets
- 2 tablespoons olive oil
- 2 tablespoons lemon juice
- 2 cloves garlic, minced
- 1 tablespoon chopped fresh parsley
- 1 tablespoon chopped fresh thyme
- Salt and pepper to taste

Instructions:

1. Preheat oven to 400°F (200°C).
2. Place flounder fillets on a baking sheet lined with parchment paper.
3. In a small bowl, whisk together olive oil, lemon juice, garlic, parsley, thyme, salt, and pepper.
4. Drizzle the mixture over the flounder fillets.
5. Bake for 15-20 minutes, or until the fish is cooked through and flakes easily with a fork.

Nutritional Information (per serving): *Calories: 250, Protein: 25g, Fat: 12g*

11. Tuna Nicoise Salad

Servings: *2* **Prep time:** *20 minutes*

Ingredients:

- 4 cups mixed greens (arugula, romaine, or spinach)
- 2 (5-ounce) cans tuna in water, drained
- 4 small red potatoes, boiled and quartered
- 1 cup green beans, trimmed and steamed
- 4 hard-boiled eggs, quartered
- ½ cup cherry tomatoes, halved
- ½ cup Kalamata olives
- 2 tablespoons chopped fresh parsley
- **Dijon Vinaigrette:**
- ¼ cup extra-virgin olive oil
- 2 tablespoons red wine vinegar
- 1 teaspoon Dijon mustard
- Salt and pepper to taste

Instructions:

1. Arrange mixed greens on a platter or individual plates.
2. Top with tuna, potatoes, green beans, eggs, tomatoes, and olives.
3. Sprinkle with parsley.

4. In a small bowl, whisk together vinaigrette ingredients.

5. Drizzle vinaigrette over salad and serve.

Nutritional Information (per serving): *Calories: 450, Protein: 30g, Fat: 28g, Fiber: 8g*

12. Shrimp Stir-Fry with Ginger and Broccoli

Servings: *2* ***Prep time:*** *15 minutes* ***Cook time:*** *15 minutes*

Ingredients:

- 1-pound large shrimp, peeled and deveined

- 1 tablespoon cornstarch

- 1 tablespoon olive oil

- 1-inch fresh ginger, grated

- 2 cloves garlic, minced

- 1 head broccoli, cut into florets

- ½ cup chopped red onion

- Stir-Fry Sauce:

- ¼ cup soy sauce (or tamari for gluten-free)

- 2 tablespoons rice vinegar

- 1 tablespoon honey

- 1 teaspoon sesame oil

- Pinch of red pepper flakes

- Cooked brown rice for serving (optional)

Instructions:

1. Toss shrimp with cornstarch.

2. Heat olive oil in a large skillet or wok over medium-high heat. Add shrimp and cook, stirring

occasionally, until pink and opaque, about 3-4 minutes per side. Remove shrimp from skillet and set aside.

3. Add ginger and garlic to the skillet and cook for 30 seconds, or until fragrant.

4. Add broccoli and red onion and cook, stirring constantly, until tender-crisp, about 5 minutes.

5. While vegetables are cooking, whisk together stir-fry sauce ingredients in a small bowl.

6. Return shrimp to the skillet and add stir-fry sauce. Cook for 1 minute more, or until heated through.

7. Serve over rice, if desired.

Nutritional Information (per serving without rice): *Calories: 320, Protein: 30g, Fat: 12g*

13. One-Pan Roasted Cod with Cherry Tomatoes and Olives

Servings: *2* ***Prep time:*** *10 minutes* ***Cook time:*** *25 minutes*

Ingredients:

- 2 (6-ounce) cod fillets
- 1-pint cherry tomatoes, halved
- ½ cup Kalamata olives, pitted
- ¼ cup chopped red onion
- 2 cloves garlic, minced
- 2 tablespoons olive oil
- ½ teaspoon dried oregano
- Salt and pepper to taste

Instructions:

1. Preheat oven to 400°F (200°C).
2. Place cod fillets on a baking sheet lined with parchment paper.
3. In a bowl, combine cherry tomatoes, olives, red onion, garlic, olive oil, oregano, salt, and pepper.
4. Spoon the tomato mixture around the cod fillets.
5. Bake for 20-25 minutes, or until fish is cooked through and flakes easily with a fork.

Nutritional Information (per serving): *Calories: 300, Protein: 28g, Fat: 16g*

14. Baked Salmon with Lemon-Dill Yogurt Sauce

***Servings:** 2 **Prep time:** 5 minutes **Cook time:** 20 minutes*

Ingredients:

- 2 (6-ounce) salmon fillets

- 1 tablespoon olive oil

- Salt and pepper to taste

- **Lemon-Dill Yogurt Sauce:**

- ½ cup plain Greek yogurt

- 2 tablespoons chopped fresh dill

- 1 tablespoon lemon juice

- Salt and pepper to taste

Instructions:

1. Preheat oven to 400°F (200°C).

2. Place salmon fillets on a baking sheet lined with parchment paper.

3. Drizzle with olive oil and season with salt and pepper.

4. Bake for 15-20 minutes, or until salmon is cooked through and flakes easily with a fork.

5. While salmon is baking, whisk together yogurt sauce ingredients in a small bowl.

6. Serve salmon with lemon-dill yogurt sauce.

***Nutritional Information (per serving):** Calories: 350, Protein: 30g, Fat: 20g*

15. Spicy Tuna Cakes with Sriracha Mayo

Servings: *2* ***Prep time:*** *15 minutes* ***Cook time:*** *10 minutes*

Ingredients:

- 2 (5-ounce) cans tuna in water, drained
- ½ cup breadcrumbs
- 1 egg, beaten
- ¼ cup chopped red onion
- ¼ cup chopped fresh cilantro
- 1 tablespoon sriracha (or other hot sauce)
- Salt and pepper to taste
- 2 tablespoons olive oil
- **Sriracha Mayo:**
- ¼ cup mayonnaise
- 1 tablespoon sriracha (or other hot sauce)

Instructions:

1. In a medium bowl, combine tuna, breadcrumbs, egg, red onion, cilantro, sriracha, salt, and pepper.

2. Form the mixture into 4 patties.

3. Heat olive oil in a large skillet over medium heat. Add tuna cakes and cook for 3-4 minutes per side, or until golden brown and cooked through.

4. While tuna cakes are cooking, whisk together mayonnaise and sriracha in a small bowl.

5. Serve tuna cakes with sriracha mayo.

Nutritional Information (per serving): *Calories: 400, Protein: 30g, Fat: 20g*

16. Mediterranean Baked Sea Bass with Fennel and Orange

Servings: *2* ***Prep time:*** *15 minutes* ***Cook time:*** *20 minutes*

Ingredients:

- 2 (6-ounce) sea bass fillets

- 1 bulb fennel, thinly sliced

- 1 orange, sliced

- 2 tablespoons olive oil

- 2 cloves garlic, minced

- 1 teaspoon fennel seeds

- Salt and pepper to taste

Instructions:

1. Preheat oven to 400°F (200°C).

2. Place fennel and orange slices on a baking sheet lined with parchment paper. Drizzle with olive oil and season with salt and pepper.

3. Roast for 10 minutes.

4. Place sea bass fillets on top of the fennel and orange slices. Sprinkle with garlic and fennel seeds. Drizzle with remaining olive oil and season with salt and pepper.

5. Bake for 10-15 minutes, or until fish is cooked through and flakes easily with a fork.

Nutritional Information (per serving): *Calories: 320, Protein: 28g, Fat: 18g*

17. Shrimp and Vegetable Skewers with Lemon Herb Marinade

Servings: *2* ***Prep time:*** *20 minutes* ***Cook time:*** *10 minutes*

Ingredients:

- 1-pound large shrimp, peeled and deveined

- 1 zucchini, cut into 1-inch chunks

- 1 red bell pepper, cut into 1-inch chunks

- 1 yellow onion, cut into 1-inch chunks

- **Lemon Herb Marinade:**

- ¼ cup olive oil

- 2 tablespoons lemon juice

- 2 cloves garlic, minced

- 1 tablespoon chopped fresh parsley

- 1 tablespoon chopped fresh oregano

- Salt and pepper to taste

Instructions:

1. Thread shrimp, zucchini, bell pepper, and onion onto skewers.

2. In a small bowl, whisk together marinade ingredients.

3. Pour marinade over skewers and toss to coat. Let marinate for at least 15 minutes.

4. Preheat grill to medium heat.

5. Grill skewers for 3-4 minutes per side, or until shrimp is pink and opaque and vegetables are tender.

Nutritional Information (per serving): Calories: 350, Protein: 30g, Fat: 18g

18. Baked Halibut with Tomato and Caper Relish

Servings: *2* ***Prep time:*** *15 minutes* ***Cook time:*** *20 minutes*

Ingredients:

- 2 (6-ounce) halibut fillets

- 1 tablespoon olive oil

- Salt and pepper to taste

- **Tomato and Caper Relish:**

- 1 cup chopped tomatoes

- ¼ cup chopped red onion

- 2 tablespoons capers

- 2 tablespoons chopped fresh parsley

- 1 tablespoon lemon juice

- Salt and pepper to taste

Instructions:

1. Preheat oven to 400°F (200°C).

2. Place halibut fillets on a baking sheet lined with parchment paper. Drizzle with olive oil and season with salt and pepper.

3. Bake for 15-20 minutes, or until fish is cooked through and flakes easily with a fork.

4. While fish is baking, combine relish ingredients in a bowl.

5. Serve halibut topped with tomato and caper relish.

Nutritional Information (per serving): *Calories: 280, Protein: 25g, Fat: 12g*

19. Asian-Inspired Tuna Salad

Servings: *2* **Prep time:** *15 minutes*

Ingredients:

- 2 (5-ounce) cans tuna in water, drained
- ½ cup shredded carrots
- ½ cup shredded red cabbage
- ¼ cup chopped red onion
- ¼ cup chopped fresh cilantro
- 2 tablespoons rice vinegar
- 1 tablespoon soy sauce (or tamari for gluten-free)
- 1 teaspoon sesame oil
- ½ teaspoon grated fresh ginger
- Pinch of red pepper flakes
- Salt and pepper to taste

Instructions:

1. In a medium bowl, combine tuna, carrots, cabbage, red onion, and cilantro.
2. In a small bowl, whisk together rice vinegar, soy sauce, sesame oil, ginger, red pepper flakes, salt, and pepper.
3. Pour the dressing over the tuna mixture and stir to combine.

4. Serve on whole-wheat bread, lettuce cups, or
   crackers.

Nutritional Information (per serving without bread): *Calories: 200, Protein: 25g, Fat: 8g*

20. Salmon Burgers with Dill Yogurt Sauce

Servings: *4* **Prep time:** *20 minutes* **Cook time:** *15 minutes*

Ingredients:

- 1-pound salmon fillet, skin removed and finely chopped
- ½ cup panko breadcrumbs
- 1 egg, beaten
- ¼ cup chopped red onion
- ¼ cup chopped fresh dill
- 1 tablespoon lemon juice
- Salt and pepper to taste
- 2 tablespoons olive oil
- **Dill Yogurt Sauce:**
- ½ cup plain Greek yogurt
- 2 tablespoons chopped fresh dill
- 1 tablespoon lemon juice
- Salt and pepper to taste
- Whole-wheat hamburger buns

Instructions:

1. In a large bowl, combine salmon, breadcrumbs, egg, red onion, dill, lemon juice, salt, and pepper.
2. Form mixture into 4 patties.
3. Heat olive oil in a large skillet over medium heat. Add salmon burgers and cook for 5-7 minutes per side, or until golden brown and cooked through.

4. While burgers are cooking, whisk together yogurt sauce ingredients in a small bowl.
5. Serve salmon burgers on whole-wheat buns with dill yogurt sauce.

Nutritional Information (per serving without bun): *Calories: 350, Protein: 30g, Fat: 20g*

The vastness of the ocean mirrors the boundless culinary possibilities that fish and seafood offer. Let this chapter be your guide to creating delicious, nutritious, and MIND-friendly meals that showcase the very best of these aquatic treasures. As you explore these 20 recipes, remember that the joy of cooking and eating is a gift to be cherished and shared with others.

Chapter 6: Poultry and Meat Mains

"A good meal is a gift to the body and the soul." This sentiment, often echoed in culinary circles, perfectly encapsulates the joy and nourishment that a well-prepared meal can bring. While the MIND diet champions the consumption of brain-healthy foods like fruits, vegetables, and whole grains, it also recognizes the value of lean protein sources, such as poultry and meat, in maintaining a balanced and satisfying diet.

In this chapter, we'll explore a delightful array of poultry and meat main dishes that adhere to the MIND diet's principles while delivering a burst of flavor and culinary creativity. You'll find recipes that showcase a variety of cooking techniques, from slow-cooking to grilling, and feature a diverse selection of herbs, spices, and seasonal vegetables.

Whether you're a seasoned home cook or a culinary novice, these recipes offer simple and accessible ways to incorporate lean protein into your meals while reaping the nutritional benefits. From comforting classics to exotic new flavors, there's something for everyone to savor and share.

1. Lemon Herb Roasted Chicken

Servings: *2* ***Prep time:*** *10 minutes* ***Cook time:*** *45 minutes*

Ingredients:

- 2 bone-in, skin-on chicken breasts
- 2 tablespoons olive oil
- 2 cloves garlic, minced
- 1 tablespoon chopped fresh rosemary
- 1 tablespoon chopped fresh thyme
- 1 lemon, zested and juiced
- Salt and pepper to taste

Instructions:

1. Preheat oven to 400°F (200°C).
2. Place chicken breasts on a baking sheet lined with parchment paper.
3. In a small bowl, combine olive oil, garlic, rosemary, thyme, lemon zest, lemon juice, salt, and pepper.
4. Rub the mixture all over the chicken breasts.
5. Bake for 40-45 minutes, or until chicken is cooked through and juices run clear.

Nutritional Information (per serving): *Calories: 350, Protein: 40g, Fat: 18g*

2. Mediterranean Chicken with Olives and Artichokes

Servings: *2* ***Prep time:*** *15 minutes* ***Cook time:*** *30 minutes*

Ingredients:

- 2 boneless, skinless chicken breasts
- 1 tablespoon olive oil
- 1 onion, chopped
- 2 cloves garlic, minced
- 1 can (14.5 ounces) diced tomatoes, undrained
- ½ cup pitted Kalamata olives
- ¼ cup marinated artichoke hearts, quartered
- ½ teaspoon dried oregano
- Salt and pepper to taste

Instructions:

1. Heat olive oil in a large skillet over medium heat. Season chicken breasts with salt and pepper.
2. Add chicken to the skillet and cook for 5-6 minutes per side, or until browned and cooked through. Remove chicken from skillet and set aside.
3. Add onion to the skillet and cook until softened, about 5 minutes.
4. Add garlic, tomatoes, olives, artichoke hearts, and oregano. Bring to a simmer and cook for 10 minutes, or until sauce thickens slightly.

5. Return chicken to the skillet and cook for 5 minutes more, or until heated through.

Nutritional Information (per serving): *Calories: 380, Protein: 35g, Fat: 18g*

3. Slow-Cooker Chicken Tikka Masala

Servings: *4* ***Prep time:*** *20 minutes* ***Cook time:*** *4-6 hours on low or 2-3 hours on high*

Ingredients:

- 2 pounds boneless, skinless chicken thighs or breasts
- 1 onion, chopped
- 3 cloves garlic, minced
- 1 tablespoon grated fresh ginger
- 2 tablespoons tikka masala paste
- 1 can (14 ounces) diced tomatoes, undrained
- 1 can (13.5 ounces) coconut milk
- ½ cup plain Greek yogurt
- 2 tablespoons chopped fresh cilantro
- Salt and pepper to taste
- Cooked brown rice or naan for serving

Instructions:

1. In a large skillet over medium heat, brown chicken in olive oil.
2. Transfer chicken to slow cooker.
3. Add onion, garlic, ginger, and tikka masala paste to the skillet and cook for 1 minute more.

4. Stir in tomatoes, coconut milk, salt, and pepper. Bring to a simmer, then pour over chicken in slow cooker.
5. Cover and cook on low for 4-6 hours or on high for 2-3 hours, or until chicken is cooked through.
6. Stir in yogurt and cilantro just before serving.
7. Serve over brown rice or with naan.

Nutritional Information (per serving): *Calories: 450, Protein: 35g, Fat: 25g*

4. Honey-Garlic Glazed Turkey Meatballs

Servings: *2* ***Prep time:*** *15 minutes* ***Cook time:*** *25 minutes*

Ingredients:

- 1-pound ground turkey
- ½ cup breadcrumbs
- ¼ cup chopped onion
- 1 egg, beaten
- 1 tablespoon chopped fresh parsley
- 1 tablespoon olive oil
- **Honey-Garlic Glaze:**
- ¼ cup honey
- 2 tablespoons soy sauce (or tamari for gluten-free)
- 2 tablespoons rice vinegar
- 1 clove garlic, minced

Instructions:

1. Preheat oven to 400°F (200°C).
2. In a large bowl, combine ground turkey, breadcrumbs, onion, egg, parsley, salt, and pepper. Mix well.
3. Form mixture into meatballs, about 1 inch in diameter.

4. Heat olive oil in a large skillet over medium heat. Add meatballs and cook, turning occasionally, until browned on all sides.
5. In a small bowl, whisk together honey-garlic glaze ingredients.
6. Transfer meatballs to a baking dish and pour glaze over them.
7. Bake for 15-20 minutes, or until cooked through.

Nutritional Information (per serving): *Calories: 400, Protein: 30g, Fat: 20g*

5. Balsamic Glazed Chicken with Roasted Brussels Sprouts and Grapes

Servings: *2* ***Prep time:*** *15 minutes* ***Cook time:*** *35 minutes*

Ingredients:

- 2 boneless, skinless chicken breasts
- 1 tablespoon olive oil
- Salt and pepper to taste
- 1-pound Brussels sprouts, trimmed and halved
- 1 cup red grapes
- **Balsamic Glaze:**
- ¼ cup balsamic vinegar
- 1 tablespoon honey
- 1 teaspoon Dijon mustard

Instructions:

1. Preheat oven to 400°F (200°C).

2. Place chicken breasts on a baking sheet lined with parchment paper. Drizzle with olive oil and season with salt and pepper.

3. In a separate bowl, toss Brussels sprouts and grapes with olive oil, salt, and pepper. Spread on a separate baking sheet.

4. Roast chicken and vegetables for 20-25 minutes, or until chicken is cooked through and vegetables are tender.

5. While chicken and vegetables are roasting, whisk together balsamic glaze ingredients in a small saucepan. Bring to a simmer and cook for 5 minutes, or until thickened.

6. Remove chicken and vegetables from oven. Drizzle balsamic glaze over chicken and serve with roasted vegetables.

Nutritional Information (per serving): *Calories: 400, Protein: 35g, Fat: 18g*

6. Lemon Herb Turkey Burgers with Tzatziki Sauce

Servings: *4* ***Prep time:*** *20 minutes* ***Cook time:*** *15 minutes*

Ingredients:

- 1-pound ground turkey
- ½ cup breadcrumbs
- ¼ cup chopped red onion
- 1 egg, beaten
- 1 tablespoon chopped fresh parsley
- 1 tablespoon chopped fresh dill
- 1 tablespoon lemon juice
- Salt and pepper to taste
- 2 tablespoons olive oil
- **Tzatziki Sauce:**
- ½ cup plain Greek yogurt
- ½ cup grated cucumber (seeds removed)
- 1 tablespoon lemon juice
- 1 tablespoon chopped fresh dill
- 1 clove garlic, minced
- Salt and pepper to taste
- Whole-wheat hamburger buns

Instructions:

1. In a large bowl, combine ground turkey, breadcrumbs, onion, egg, parsley, dill, lemon juice, salt, and pepper. Mix well.

2. Form mixture into 4 patties.
3. Heat olive oil in a large skillet over medium heat. Add turkey burgers and cook for 5-7 minutes per side, or until cooked through.
4. While burgers are cooking, prepare tzatziki sauce by combining all ingredients in a bowl.
5. Serve turkey burgers on whole-wheat buns with tzatziki sauce.

Nutritional Information (per serving without bun): *Calories: 350, Protein: 30g, Fat: 18g*

7. Chicken Piccata with Lemon Caper Sauce

Servings: *2* **Prep time:** *15 minutes* **Cook time:** *20 minutes*

Ingredients:

- 2 boneless, skinless chicken breasts
- ½ cup all-purpose flour
- Salt and pepper to taste
- 2 tablespoons olive oil
- 2 tablespoons butter
- ½ cup chicken broth
- ¼ cup lemon juice
- 2 tablespoons capers
- 1 tablespoon chopped fresh parsley

Instructions:

1. Dredge chicken breasts in flour seasoned with salt and pepper.
2. Heat olive oil and butter in a large skillet over medium heat.
3. Add chicken breasts and cook for 5-6 minutes per side, or until golden brown and cooked through. Remove chicken from skillet and set aside.

4. Add chicken broth and lemon juice to the skillet. Bring to a simmer and cook for 2 minutes, or until slightly reduced.

5. Stir in capers and parsley.

6. Return chicken to the skillet and cook for 1 minute more, or until heated through.

Nutritional Information (per serving): *Calories: 400, Protein: 35g, Fat: 20g*

8. Apricot Glazed Chicken with Roasted Vegetables

Servings: *2* ***Prep time:*** *15 minutes* ***Cook time:*** *35 minutes*

Ingredients:

- 2 boneless, skinless chicken breasts
- 1 tablespoon olive oil
- Salt and pepper to taste
- 1 cup diced butternut squash
- 1 cup Brussels sprouts, trimmed and halved
- ½ cup red onion, cut into wedges
- **Apricot Glaze:**
- ¼ cup apricot preserves
- 2 tablespoons Dijon mustard
- 1 tablespoon apple cider vinegar

Instructions:

1. Preheat oven to 400°F (200°C).
2. Place chicken breasts on a baking sheet lined with parchment paper. Drizzle with olive oil and season with salt and pepper.
3. In a separate bowl, toss butternut squash, Brussels sprouts, and red onion with olive oil,

salt, and pepper. Spread on a separate baking sheet.

4. Roast chicken and vegetables for 20-25 minutes, or until chicken is cooked through and vegetables are tender.

5. While chicken and vegetables are roasting, whisk together apricot glaze ingredients in a small bowl.

6. Brush glaze over chicken during the last 5 minutes of cooking time.

7. Serve chicken with roasted vegetables.

Nutritional Information (per serving): *Calories: 450, Protein: 35g, Fat: 20g*

9. One-Pan Chicken with Roasted Root Vegetables and Rosemary

*Servings: 2 **Prep time:** 15 minutes **Cook time:** 45 minutes*

Ingredients:

- 2 bone-in, skin-on chicken thighs
- 1 sweet potato, peeled and cubed
- 2 carrots, peeled and cut into chunks
- 1 parsnip, peeled and cut into chunks
- 1 red onion, cut into wedges
- 2 tablespoons olive oil
- 2 sprigs fresh rosemary
- Salt and pepper to taste

Instructions:

1. Preheat oven to 400°F (200°C).
2. Place chicken thighs and vegetables on a baking sheet lined with parchment paper.
3. Drizzle with olive oil and sprinkle with rosemary, salt, and pepper.
4. Roast for 40-45 minutes, or until chicken is cooked through and vegetables are tender.

Nutritional Information (per serving): *Calories: 400, Protein: 30g, Fat: 20g*

10. Turmeric-Roasted Chicken with Chickpeas and Vegetables

Servings: *2* ***Prep time:*** *15 minutes* ***Cook time:*** *40 minutes*

Ingredients:

- 2 boneless, skinless chicken breasts
- 1 tablespoon olive oil
- 1 teaspoon ground turmeric
- ½ teaspoon ground cumin
- ½ teaspoon ground coriander
- Salt and pepper to taste
- 1 can (15 ounces) chickpeas, rinsed and drained
- 1 sweet potato, peeled and cubed
- 1 red onion, cut into wedges
- ¼ cup chopped fresh cilantro

Instructions:

1. Preheat oven to 400°F (200°C).
2. Place chicken breasts on a baking sheet lined with parchment paper.
3. In a small bowl, combine olive oil, turmeric, cumin, coriander, salt, and pepper.
4. Rub the mixture all over the chicken breasts.

5. Add chickpeas, sweet potato, and red onion to the baking sheet. Drizzle with olive oil and season with salt and pepper.

6. Roast for 30-35 minutes, or until chicken is cooked through and vegetables are tender.

7. Sprinkle with cilantro before serving.

Nutritional Information (per serving): *Calories: 450, Protein: 35g, Fat: 18g*

11. Sheet Pan Chicken Fajitas

Servings: *4* **Prep time:** *15 minutes* **Cook time:** *25 minutes*

Ingredients:

- 1 pound boneless, skinless chicken breasts, sliced
- 1 bell pepper (any color), sliced
- 1 onion, sliced
- 1 tablespoon olive oil
- 1 tablespoon fajita seasoning
- Salt and pepper to taste
- Whole-wheat tortillas
- Optional toppings: avocado, salsa, guacamole, shredded lettuce, chopped tomatoes

Instructions:

1. Preheat oven to 400°F (200°C).
2. In a large bowl, toss chicken, bell pepper, and onion with olive oil, fajita seasoning, salt, and pepper.
3. Spread the mixture in a single layer on a baking sheet lined with parchment paper.

4. Roast for 20-25 minutes, or until chicken is cooked through and vegetables are tender.

5. Warm tortillas in a dry skillet or microwave.

6. Fill tortillas with chicken and vegetable mixture and desired toppings.

Nutritional Information (per serving without toppings): *Calories: 300, Protein: 25g, Fat: 10g*

12. Chicken and Vegetable Curry

Servings: *4* ***Prep time:*** *15 minutes* ***Cook time:*** *30 minutes*

Ingredients:

- 1 tablespoon olive oil
- 1 onion, chopped
- 2 cloves garlic, minced
- 1 tablespoon curry powder
- ½ teaspoon ground ginger
- 1-pound boneless, skinless chicken breasts, cut into 1-inch pieces
- 1 sweet potato, peeled and diced
- 1 head broccoli, cut into florets
- 1 can (14 ounces) coconut milk
- ½ cup chicken broth
- Salt and pepper to taste
- Cooked brown rice or quinoa for serving

Instructions:

1. Heat olive oil in a large pot or Dutch oven over medium heat. Add onion and cook until softened, about 5 minutes.
2. Add garlic, curry powder, and ginger and cook for 1 minute more.

3. Add chicken and cook until browned on all sides.

4. Stir in sweet potato, broccoli, coconut milk, and broth. Bring to a boil, then reduce heat and simmer for 20 minutes, or until chicken is cooked through and vegetables are tender.

5. Season with salt and pepper to taste.

6. Serve over brown rice or quinoa.

Nutritional Information (per serving): *Calories: 400, Protein: 30g, Fat: 18g*

13. Lemon Herb Turkey Burgers

Servings: *4* ***Prep time:*** *15 minutes* ***Cook time:*** *10 minutes*

Ingredients:

- 1-pound ground turkey
- ½ cup panko breadcrumbs
- 1 egg, beaten
- ¼ cup chopped red onion
- 1 tablespoon chopped fresh parsley
- 1 tablespoon chopped fresh dill
- 1 tablespoon lemon juice
- Salt and pepper to taste
- 2 tablespoons olive oil
- Whole-wheat hamburger buns
- Optional toppings: avocado, lettuce, tomato, red onion

Instructions:

1. In a large bowl, combine ground turkey, breadcrumbs, egg, onion, parsley, dill, lemon juice, salt, and pepper. Mix well.
2. Form mixture into 4 patties.
3. Heat olive oil in a large skillet over medium heat. Add turkey burgers and cook for 5-7 minutes per side, or until cooked through.
4. Serve on whole-wheat buns with desired toppings.

Nutritional Information (per serving without bun): *Calories: 250, Protein: 25g, Fat: 12g*

14. Chicken and White Bean Stew with Kale and Lemon

Servings: *2* ***Prep time:*** *15 minutes* ***Cook time:*** *30 minutes*

Ingredients:

- 1 tablespoon olive oil
- 1 onion, chopped
- 2 cloves garlic, minced
- 1 teaspoon dried oregano
- ½ teaspoon dried thyme
- Pinch of red pepper flakes
- 1-pound boneless, skinless chicken breasts, cut into 1-inch pieces
- 1 can (15 ounces) cannellini beans, rinsed and drained
- 4 cups chicken broth
- 2 cups chopped kale
- 1 lemon, zested and juiced
- Salt and pepper to taste

Instructions:

1. Heat olive oil in a large pot or Dutch oven over medium heat.

2. Add onion and cook until softened, about 5 minutes.

3. Add garlic, oregano, thyme, and red pepper flakes and cook for 1 minute more.

4. Add chicken and cook until browned on all sides.

5. Stir in beans, broth, kale, lemon zest, and lemon juice. Bring to a boil, then reduce heat and simmer for 15 minutes, or until chicken is cooked through and kale is tender.

6. Season with salt and pepper to taste.

Nutritional Information (per serving): *Calories: 400, Protein: 35g, Fat: 15g, Fiber: 10g*

15. Greek Chicken Kabobs with Tzatziki Sauce

Servings: *2* ***Prep time:*** *20 minutes* ***Cook time:*** *15 minutes*

Ingredients:

- 1-pound boneless, skinless chicken breasts, cut into 1-inch cubes
- ½ red onion, cut into chunks
- 1 green bell pepper, cut into chunks
- 10 cherry tomatoes
- **Greek Marinade:**
- ¼ cup olive oil
- 2 tablespoons lemon juice
- 2 cloves garlic, minced
- 1 teaspoon dried oregano
- Salt and pepper to taste
- **Tzatziki Sauce:**
- ½ cup plain Greek yogurt
- ½ cup grated cucumber (seeds removed)
- 1 tablespoon lemon juice
- 1 tablespoon chopped fresh dill
- 1 clove garlic, minced
- Salt and pepper to taste

1. In a large bowl, combine chicken, onion, bell pepper, and tomatoes.
2. In a small bowl, whisk together marinade ingredients.
3. Pour marinade over chicken and vegetables and toss to coat. Let marinate for at least 15 minutes.
4. Preheat grill or broiler to medium heat.
5. Thread chicken and vegetables onto skewers.
6. Grill or broil for 10-12 minutes, or until chicken is cooked through and vegetables are tender.
7. While skewers are cooking, prepare tzatziki sauce by combining all ingredients in a bowl.
8. Serve skewers with tzatziki sauce.

Nutritional Information (per serving): *Calories: 380, Protein: 35g, Fat: 20g*

16. Chicken Stir-Fry with Broccoli and Cashews

Servings: *2* ***Prep time:*** *15 minutes* ***Cook time:*** *20 minutes*

Ingredients:

- 1-pound boneless, skinless chicken breasts, sliced
- 1 tablespoon cornstarch
- 1 tablespoon olive oil
- 1 head broccoli, cut into florets
- ½ cup chopped red onion
- ¼ cup chopped cashews
- **Stir-Fry Sauce:**
- ¼ cup soy sauce (or tamari for gluten-free)
- 2 tablespoons rice vinegar
- 1 tablespoon honey
- 1 teaspoon sesame oil
- Pinch of red pepper flakes
- Cooked brown rice or noodles for serving (optional)

Instructions:

1. Toss chicken with cornstarch.

2. Heat olive oil in a large skillet or wok over medium-high heat. Add chicken and cook, stirring occasionally, until browned on all sides. Remove chicken from skillet and set aside.

3. Add broccoli and red onion to the skillet and cook, stirring constantly, until tender-crisp, about 5 minutes.

4. While vegetables are cooking, whisk together stir-fry sauce ingredients in a small bowl.

5. Return chicken to the skillet and add stir-fry sauce. Cook for 1 minute more, or until heated through.

6. Sprinkle with cashews and serve over rice or noodles, if desired.

Nutritional Information (per serving without rice or noodles): *Calories: 350, Protein: 30g, Fat: 15g*

17. Honey Mustard Chicken with Roasted Vegetables

Servings: *2* ***Prep time:*** *10 minutes* ***Cook time:*** *30 minutes*

Ingredients:

- 2 boneless, skinless chicken breasts
- 1 tablespoon olive oil
- Salt and pepper to taste
- 1 cup diced butternut squash
- 1 cup Brussels sprouts, trimmed and halved
- ½ cup red onion, cut into wedges
- **Honey Mustard Sauce:**
- ¼ cup Dijon mustard
- 2 tablespoons honey
- 1 tablespoon apple cider vinegar

Instructions:

1. Preheat oven to 400°F (200°C).
2. Place chicken breasts on a baking sheet lined with parchment paper. Drizzle with olive oil and season with salt and pepper.
3. In a separate bowl, toss butternut squash, Brussels sprouts, and red onion with olive oil,

salt, and pepper. Spread on a separate baking sheet.

4. Roast chicken and vegetables for 20-25 minutes, or until chicken is cooked through and vegetables are tender.
5. While chicken and vegetables are roasting, whisk together honey mustard sauce ingredients in a small bowl.
6. Serve chicken with roasted vegetables and honey mustard sauce.

Nutritional Information (per serving): *Calories: 400, Protein: 35g, Fat: 18g*

18. Moroccan Turkey Tagine with Apricots and Prunes

Servings: *4* **Prep time:** *20 minutes* **Cook time:** *45 minutes*

Ingredients:

- 1 tablespoon olive oil
- 1 onion, chopped
- 2 cloves garlic, minced
- 1 teaspoon ground cumin
- 1 teaspoon ground coriander
- ½ teaspoon turmeric
- ¼ teaspoon cinnamon
- Pinch of cayenne pepper (optional)
- 1-pound ground turkey
- 1 can (14.5 ounces) diced tomatoes, undrained
- ½ cup dried apricots, chopped
- ½ cup pitted prunes, chopped
- 1 cup chicken broth
- ½ cup chopped fresh cilantro
- Salt and pepper to taste
- Cooked couscous for serving

Instructions:

1. Heat olive oil in a large pot or Dutch oven over medium heat. Add onion and cook until softened, about 5 minutes.

2. Add garlic, cumin, coriander, turmeric, cinnamon, and cayenne pepper (if using) and cook for 1 minute more.
3. Add ground turkey and cook, breaking up with a spoon, until browned.
4. Stir in tomatoes, apricots, prunes, and broth. Bring to a boil, then reduce heat and simmer for 30 minutes, or until flavors meld and sauce thickens slightly.
5. Stir in cilantro and season with salt and pepper to taste.
6. Serve over couscous.

Nutritional Information (per serving): *Calories: 420, Protein: 28g, Fat: 15g*

19. Chicken Stir-Fry with Snow Peas and Mushrooms

Servings: *2* ***Prep time****: 15 minutes* ***Cook time:*** *20 minutes*

Ingredients:

- 1-pound boneless, skinless chicken breasts, sliced
- 1 tablespoon cornstarch
- 1 tablespoon olive oil
- 8 ounces mushrooms, sliced
- 1 cup snow peas, trimmed
- 1 red bell pepper, sliced
- 2 cloves garlic, minced
- **Stir-Fry Sauce:**
- ¼ cup soy sauce (or tamari for gluten-free)
- 2 tablespoons rice vinegar
- 1 tablespoon honey
- 1 teaspoon sesame oil
- Pinch of red pepper flakes
- Cooked brown rice or noodles for serving (optional)

Instructions:

1. Toss chicken with cornstarch.

2. Heat olive oil in a large skillet or wok over medium-high heat. Add chicken and cook, stirring occasionally, until browned on all sides. Remove chicken from skillet and set aside.

3. Add mushrooms, snow peas, bell pepper, and garlic to the skillet and cook, stirring constantly, until vegetables are tender-crisp, about 5 minutes.

4. While vegetables are cooking, whisk together stir-fry sauce ingredients in a small bowl.

5. Return chicken to the skillet and add stir-fry sauce. Cook for 1 minute more, or until heated through.

6. Serve over rice or noodles, if desired.

Nutritional Information (per serving without rice or noodles): *Calories: 350, Protein: 30g, Fat: 15g*

20. Chicken and Vegetable Skewers with Peanut Sauce

Servings: *2* ***Prep time:*** *20 minutes* ***Cook time:*** *10 minutes*

Ingredients:

- 1-pound boneless, skinless chicken breasts, cut into 1-inch cubes
- 1 red onion, cut into chunks
- 1 green bell pepper, cut into chunks
- 1 yellow squash, cut into chunks
- **Peanut Marinade:**
  - ¼ cup peanut butter
  - 2 tablespoons soy sauce (or tamari for gluten-free)
  - 2 tablespoons lime juice
  - 1 tablespoon honey
  - 1 teaspoon grated fresh ginger
  - Pinch of red pepper flakes

Instructions:

1. Thread chicken, onion, bell pepper, and squash onto skewers.
2. In a small bowl, whisk together marinade ingredients.

3. Pour marinade over skewers and toss to coat. Let marinate for at least 15 minutes.
4. Preheat grill to medium heat.
5. Grill skewers for 8-10 minutes, or until chicken is cooked through and vegetables are tender.

Nutritional Information (per serving): *Calories: 400, Protein: 30g, Fat: 22g*

With these 20 poultry and meat main dishes, you have a wealth of flavorful and healthy options to explore within the MIND diet. Remember, moderation is key when it comes to these protein sources, but with a bit of creativity and culinary curiosity, you can easily incorporate them into your weekly meal rotation while reaping their nutritional benefits.

Chapter 7: Snacks and Sweet Treats

"Life is uncertain. Eat dessert first." This playful adage, often attributed to Ernestine Ulmer, reminds us to embrace life's simple pleasures, and what better way to do so than with a delectable treat? While maintaining a balanced diet is crucial for overall health, indulging in the occasional sweet treat can bring joy and satisfaction, especially when those treats are crafted with wholesome ingredients and align with the principles of the MIND diet.

This chapter is a celebration of snacks and sweet treats that nourish both body and soul. We'll explore a diverse range of options, from savory bites packed with protein and fiber to guilt-free desserts that satisfy your sweet tooth without derailing your health goals. By focusing on whole, unprocessed ingredients and mindful portions, you can enjoy these treats as part of a balanced MIND diet lifestyle.

1. Spiced Nuts and Seeds

*Servings: 4 **Prep time:** 5 minutes **Cook time:** 15 minutes*

Ingredients:

- 1 cup raw almonds
- 1 cup raw walnuts
- ½ cup pumpkin seeds
- ½ cup sunflower seeds
- 1 tablespoon olive oil
- 1 teaspoon cumin
- ½ teaspoon paprika
- ¼ teaspoon cayenne pepper
- ½ teaspoon salt

Instructions:

1. Preheat oven to 350°F (175°C).
2. In a large bowl, combine nuts, seeds, olive oil, cumin, paprika, cayenne pepper, and salt.
3. Spread the mixture on a baking sheet and bake for 15 minutes, or until toasted and fragrant.
4. Let cool completely before storing in an airtight container.

Nutritional Information (per serving): *Calories: 200, Protein: 8g, Fat: 17g, Fiber: 4g*

2. Dark Chocolate Almond Bark

*Servings: 8 **Prep time:** 10 minutes **Chill time:** 30 minutes*

Ingredients:

- 8 ounces dark chocolate (70% cocoa or higher), chopped
- ½ cup sliced almonds

Instructions:

1. Line a baking sheet with parchment paper.
2. Melt chocolate in a double boiler or microwave-safe bowl.
3. Spread melted chocolate in an even layer on the prepared baking sheet.
4. Sprinkle almonds evenly over the chocolate.
5. Refrigerate for 30 minutes, or until chocolate is set.
6. Break into pieces and enjoy.

***Nutritional Information (per serving):** Calories: 150, Protein: 3g, Fat: 12g*

Servings: 1 **Prep time:** 5 minutes

Ingredients:

- ½ cup plain Greek yogurt

- ½ cup mixed berries

- 2 tablespoons granola

Instructions:

1. Layer yogurt, berries, and granola in a glass or bowl.

2. Repeat layers as desired.

3. Enjoy immediately.

Nutritional Information: Calories: 200, Protein: 10g, Fat: 5g, Fiber: 6g

4. Fruit Salad with Honey-Lime Dressing

Servings: *4* ***Prep time:*** *15 minutes*

Ingredients:

- 2 cups mixed fruits (berries, melon, grapes, oranges)

- 2 tablespoons honey

- 2 tablespoons lime juice

- 1 tablespoon chopped fresh mint

Instructions:

1. In a large bowl, combine fruits.

2. In a small bowl, whisk together honey, lime juice, and mint.

3. Pour dressing over fruit and toss to coat.

4. Serve chilled.

Nutritional Information (per serving): *Calories: 100, Protein: 1g, Fat: 0g, Fiber: 4g*

5. Avocado and Egg Salad

Servings: *2* ***Prep time:*** *10 minutes*

Ingredients:

- 1 avocado, mashed

- 2 hard-boiled eggs, chopped

- 2 tablespoons chopped red onion

- 2 tablespoons chopped fresh dill

- 1 tablespoon lemon juice

- Salt and pepper to taste

Instructions:

1. In a medium bowl, combine avocado, eggs, red onion, dill, lemon juice, salt, and pepper.

2. Mash with a fork until combined.

3. Serve on whole-wheat bread, lettuce cups, or crackers.

Nutritional Information (per serving): *Calories: 250, Protein: 12g, Fat: 18g*

6. Hummus and Veggie Sticks

Servings: *2* ***Prep time:*** *5 minutes*

Ingredients:

- ½ cup hummus

- Assorted vegetables for dipping (carrots, celery, cucumber, bell peppers)

Instructions:

1. Arrange vegetables on a platter.

2. Serve with hummus for dipping.

Nutritional Information (per serving): *Calories: 200, Protein: 5g, Fat: 12g, Fiber: 8g*

7. Apple Slices with Almond Butter

Servings: *1* ***Prep time:*** *5 minutes*

Ingredients:

- 1 apple, sliced

- 2 tablespoons almond butter

Instructions:

1. Spread almond butter on apple slices.

2. Enjoy!

Nutritional Information: *Calories: 200, Protein: 6g, Fat: 14g, Fiber: 5g*

8. Watermelon and Feta Bites

Servings: *4* **Prep time:** *10 minutes*

Ingredients:

- 1 cup cubed watermelon

- ¼ cup crumbled feta cheese

- ¼ cup chopped fresh mint

Instructions:

1. Thread watermelon, feta, and mint onto toothpicks or skewers.

Nutritional Information (per serving): *Calories: 50, Protein: 2g, Fat: 2g*

9. Edamame with Sea Salt

Servings: *1* ***Prep time:*** *5 minutes* ***Cook time:*** *5 minutes*

Ingredients:

- 1 cup frozen shelled edamame

- ¼ teaspoon sea salt

Instructions:

1. Steam or boil edamame according to package directions.

2. Drain and sprinkle with sea salt.

Nutritional Information: *Calories: 120, Protein: 12g, Fat: 5g, Fiber: 8g*

10. Spiced Apple Chips

Servings: *2* ***Prep time:*** *5 minutes* ***Cook time:*** *2 hours*

Ingredients:

- 2 apples, thinly sliced
- ½ teaspoon cinnamon
- ¼ teaspoon nutmeg

Instructions:

1. Preheat oven to 200°F (95°C).

2. Line baking sheets with parchment paper.

3. Toss apple slices with cinnamon and nutmeg.

4. Arrange apple slices in a single layer on the prepared baking sheets.

5. Bake for 2 hours, or until crisp, flipping halfway through.

Nutritional Information (per serving): *Calories: 80, Protein: 0g, Fat: 0g, Fiber: 4g*

11. Frozen Yogurt Bark with Berries and Granola

Servings: *4* ***Prep time:*** *10 minutes* ***Freeze time:*** *2 hours*

Ingredients:

- 2 cups plain Greek yogurt
- ¼ cup honey
- 1 cup mixed berries
- ½ cup granola

Instructions:

1. Line a baking sheet with parchment paper.
2. In a medium bowl, stir together yogurt and honey.
3. Spread yogurt mixture evenly on the prepared baking sheet.
4. Top with berries and granola.
5. Freeze for at least 2 hours, or until firm.
6. Break into pieces and enjoy.

Nutritional Information (per serving): *Calories: 150, Protein: 8g, Fat: 3g, Fiber: 3g*

12. Chocolate Avocado Mousse

Servings: *2* ***Prep time:*** *10 minutes* ***Chill time:*** *30 minutes*

Ingredients:

- 1 ripe avocado
- ¼ cup unsweetened cocoa powder
- ¼ cup maple syrup or honey
- 2 tablespoons almond milk
- ½ teaspoon vanilla extract
- Pinch of salt

Instructions:

1. In a food processor or blender, combine all ingredients.
2. Process until smooth and creamy.
3. Divide among two small bowls or ramekins.
4. Refrigerate for at least 30 minutes before serving.

Nutritional Information (per serving): *Calories: 250, Protein: 4g, Fat: 18g, Fiber: 10g*

13. Energy Bites with Dates and Oats

Servings: *12* ***Prep time:*** *15 minutes* ***Chill time:***

30 minutes

Ingredients:

- 1 cup pitted dates
- ½ cup rolled oats
- ¼ cup almond butter
- ¼ cup shredded coconut
- ¼ cup chopped nuts (almonds, walnuts, or pecans)
- 2 tablespoons chia seeds
- 1 tablespoon water

Instructions:

1. In a food processor, combine dates, oats, almond butter, coconut, nuts, and chia seeds.
2. Pulse until a sticky dough form.
3. Add water 1 tablespoon at a time, pulsing until the mixture holds together.
4. Roll dough into 1-inch balls.
5. Refrigerate for 30 minutes before serving.

Nutritional Information (per serving): *Calories: 100, Protein: 2g, Fat: 5g, Fiber: 3g*

14. Roasted Chickpeas with Lemon and Herbs

Servings: *2* ***Prep time:*** *5 minutes* ***Cook time:*** *30 minutes*

Ingredients:

- 1 can (15 ounces) chickpeas, rinsed, drained, and patted dry
- 1 tablespoon olive oil
- 1 teaspoon dried oregano
- ½ teaspoon dried thyme
- ½ teaspoon garlic powder
- ½ teaspoon salt
- ¼ teaspoon black pepper
- Zest of 1 lemon

Instructions:

1. Preheat oven to 400°F (200°C).
2. In a bowl, toss chickpeas with olive oil, oregano, thyme, garlic powder, salt, pepper, and lemon zest.
3. Spread chickpeas in a single layer on a baking sheet.
4. Bake for 30 minutes, or until golden brown and crispy.

Nutritional Information (per serving): *Calories: 180, Protein: 7g, Fat: 6g, Fiber: 7g*

15. Baked Pears with Cinnamon and Honey

Servings: *2* ***Prep time:*** *5 minutes* ***Cook time:*** *20 minutes*

Ingredients:

- 2 pears, halved and cored
- 1 tablespoon honey
- 1 teaspoon cinnamon
- Pinch of nutmeg

Instructions:

1. Preheat oven to 350°F (175°C).
2. Place pears cut-side up in a baking dish.
3. Drizzle with honey and sprinkle with cinnamon and nutmeg.
4. Bake for 20-25 minutes, or until tender.
5. Serve warm or at room temperature.

Nutritional Information (per serving): *Calories: 120, Protein: 1g, Fat: 0g, Fiber: 5g*

16. Frozen Banana Bites with Peanut Butter and Chocolate

Servings: *4* **Prep time:** *10 minutes* **Freeze time**: *1 hour*

- 2 bananas, sliced

- ¼ cup peanut butter

- 2 ounces dark chocolate (70% cocoa or higher), melted

1. Spread peanut butter on half of the banana slices.

2. Top with remaining banana slices to make sandwiches.

3. Dip each sandwich in melted chocolate and place on a parchment-lined baking sheet.

4. Freeze for at least 1 hour, or until chocolate is set.

Nutritional Information (per serving): *Calories: 180, Protein: 4g, Fat: 10g*

17. Greek Yogurt with Berries and Honey

Servings: *1* **Prep time:** *5 minutes*

Ingredients:

- ½ cup plain Greek yogurt

- ½ cup mixed berries

- 1 tablespoon honey

Instructions:

1. In a bowl, combine yogurt and honey.

2. Top with berries.

Nutritional Information: *Calories: 150, Protein: 12g, Fat: 3g, Fiber: 4g*

18. Ants on a Log

Servings: *2* ***Prep time:*** *5 minutes*

Ingredients:

- 2 stalks celery, cut into 4-inch pieces
- 2 tablespoons peanut butter
- ¼ cup raisins

Instructions:

1. Fill celery stalks with peanut butter.
2. Top with raisins.

Nutritional Information (per serving): *Calories: 150, Protein: 5g, Fat: 9g, Fiber: 3g*

19. Banana Nice Cream

***Servings:** 1 **Prep time:** 5 minutes **Freeze time:** 2 hours*

Ingredients:

- 2 frozen bananas

Instructions:

1. Freeze bananas for at least 2 hours.

2. Place frozen bananas in a food processor or blender and process until smooth and creamy.

***Nutritional Information:** Calories: 105, Protein: 1g, Fat: 0g, Fiber: 3g*

20. Fruit and Cheese Plate

***Servings:** 2 **Prep time:** 10 minutes*

Ingredients:

- ½ cup grapes

- ½ apple, sliced

- ¼ cup berries

- 2 ounces cheese (cheddar, mozzarella, or feta)

- 2 whole-wheat crackers

Instructions:

1. Arrange fruit and cheese on a plate.

2. Serve with crackers.

***Nutritional Information (per serving):** Calories: 200, Protein: 10g, Fat: 12g*

This chapter is a testament to the fact that healthy snacks and sweet treats can be just as satisfying and delicious as their less healthy counterparts. By choosing whole, unprocessed ingredients and incorporating plenty of fruits, vegetables, and nuts, you can enjoy a wide variety of snacks and desserts that align with the MIND diet principles. Remember, moderation is key, but don't be afraid to indulge in the occasional treat – it's all part of a balanced and healthy lifestyle.

Chapter 8: Dressings and Sauces

"A sauce can save a dish...or kill it." This culinary adage, often echoed in kitchens around the world, speaks to the transformative power of dressings and sauces. These seemingly simple additions have the ability to elevate a meal from ordinary to extraordinary, infusing it with layers of flavor, texture, and aroma. In the context of the MIND diet, dressings and sauces not only enhance the palatability of our dishes but also contribute valuable nutrients and antioxidants.

This chapter invites you to explore a vibrant collection of 20 dressings and sauce recipes that align perfectly with the MIND diet's principles. You'll find options that span a spectrum of flavors, from tangy and zesty to creamy and savory. Each recipe is crafted with wholesome ingredients like olive oil, herbs, spices, nuts, seeds, and fresh produce, ensuring that every drizzle or dollop not only delights your taste buds but also nourishes your body and brain.

Whether you're dressing a salad, drizzling it over grilled vegetables, or using it as a dip for your favorite snacks, these versatile dressings and sauces will add a touch of culinary magic to your MIND diet meals.

1. Lemon-Tahini Dressing

Yields: *1 cup* **Prep time:** *5 minutes*

Ingredients:

- ¼ cup tahini

- ¼ cup water

- 2 tablespoons lemon juice

- 2 tablespoons extra-virgin olive oil

- 1 clove garlic, minced

- 1 tablespoon chopped fresh parsley

- Salt and pepper to taste

Instructions:

1. In a small bowl, whisk together tahini, water, lemon juice, olive oil, garlic, parsley, salt, and pepper until smooth and creamy.

2. Adjust consistency with additional water if needed.

Nutritional Information (per 2 tbsp serving):

Calories: 100, Protein: 3g, Fat: 9g, Carbohydrates: 2g

2. Creamy Avocado Dressing

Yields: *1 cup* ***Prep time:*** *5 minutes*

Ingredients:

- 1 ripe avocado, pitted and peeled
- ¼ cup plain Greek yogurt
- 2 tablespoons lime juice
- 2 tablespoons water
- 1 tablespoon chopped fresh cilantro
- Salt and pepper to taste

Instructions:

1. In a food processor or blender, combine avocado, yogurt, lime juice, water, cilantro, salt, and pepper.
2. Blend until smooth and creamy.

Nutritional Information (per 2 tbsp serving):

Calories: 60, Protein: 1g, Fat: 5g, Carbohydrates: 2g

3. Honey Mustard Vinaigrette

Yields: *½ cup* ***Prep time:*** *5 minutes*

Ingredients:

- ¼ cup extra-virgin olive oil

- 2 tablespoons Dijon mustard

- 2 tablespoons apple cider vinegar

- 1 tablespoon honey

- 1 teaspoon minced shallot

- Salt and pepper to taste

Instructions:

1. In a small bowl, whisk together olive oil, Dijon mustard, apple cider vinegar, honey, shallot, salt, and pepper until emulsified.

Nutritional Information (per 2 tbsp serving):
Calories: 120, Protein: 0g, Fat: 12g, Carbohydrates: 2g

4. Balsamic Vinaigrette

Yields: *½ cup* ***Prep time:*** *5 minutes*

Ingredients:

- ¼ cup balsamic vinegar

- ¼ cup extra-virgin olive oil

- 1 teaspoon Dijon mustard

- 1 clove garlic, minced

- Salt and pepper to taste

Instructions:

1. In a small bowl, whisk together balsamic vinegar, olive oil, Dijon mustard, garlic, salt, and pepper until emulsified.

Nutritional Information (per 2 tbsp serving):
Calories: 120, Protein: 0g, Fat: 12g, Carbohydrates: 2g

5. Raspberry Vinaigrette

Yields: *½ cup* ***Prep time:*** *5 minutes*

Ingredients:

- ¼ cup raspberries

- 2 tablespoons extra-virgin olive oil

- 2 tablespoons red wine vinegar

- 1 tablespoon honey

- Salt and pepper to taste

Instructions:

1. In a blender or food processor, combine raspberries, olive oil, red wine vinegar, honey, salt, and pepper.

2. Blend until smooth.

Nutritional Information (per 2 tbsp serving):
Calories: 80, Protein: 0g, Fat: 7g, Carbohydrates: 3g

6. Green Goddess Dressing

Yields: *1 cup* **Prep time:** *10 minutes*

Ingredients:

- 1 cup packed fresh herbs (parsley, chives, tarragon)
- 2 anchovy fillets (optional)
- 2 tablespoons mayonnaise
- 2 tablespoons lemon juice
- 2 tablespoons extra-virgin olive oil
- 1 clove garlic, minced
- Salt and pepper to taste

Instructions:

1. In a food processor or blender, combine herbs, anchovies (if using), mayonnaise, lemon juice, olive oil, garlic, salt, and pepper.
2. Blend until smooth and creamy.

Nutritional Information (per 2 tbsp serving):

Calories: 80, Protein: 1g, Fat: 8g, Carbohydrates: 1g

7. Creamy Cilantro Lime Dressing

Yields: *1 cup* ***Prep time:*** *5 minutes*

Ingredients:

- ½ cup plain Greek yogurt

- ¼ cup chopped fresh cilantro

- 2 tablespoons lime juice

- 2 tablespoons extra-virgin olive oil

- 1 clove garlic, minced

- Salt and pepper to taste

Instructions:

1. In a small bowl, whisk together yogurt, cilantro, lime juice, olive oil, garlic, salt, and pepper.

Nutritional Information (per 2 tbsp serving):
Calories: 60, Protein: 2g, Fat: 5g, Carbohydrates: 1g

8. Basil Pesto

Yields: *1 cup* ***Prep time:*** *10 minutes*

Ingredients:

- 2 cups packed fresh basil leaves

- ¼ cup pine nuts (or walnuts)

- ¼ cup grated Parmesan cheese

- 2 cloves garlic, minced

- ¼ cup extra-virgin olive oil

- Salt and pepper to taste

Instructions:

1. In a food processor or blender, combine basil, pine nuts, Parmesan, garlic, salt, and pepper.

2. Pulse until finely chopped.

3. With the motor running, drizzle in olive oil until desired consistency is reached.

Nutritional Information (per 2 tbsp serving):
Calories: 120, Protein: 2g, Fat: 12g, Carbohydrates: 1g

9. Creamy Pesto Dressing

Yields: *1 cup* **Prep time:** *5 minutes*

Ingredients:

- ½ cup prepared basil pesto (see recipe above)

- ½ cup plain Greek yogurt

- 1 tablespoon lemon juice

- Salt and pepper to taste

Instructions:

1. In a small bowl, whisk together pesto, yogurt, lemon juice, salt, and pepper.

Nutritional Information (per 2 tbsp serving):

Calories: 100, Protein: 3g, Fat: 9g, Carbohydrates: 2g

10. Sun-Dried Tomato Vinaigrette

Yields: *½ cup* ***Prep time:*** *10 minutes*

Ingredients:

- ¼ cup sun-dried tomatoes, packed in oil, drained and chopped

- 2 tablespoons extra-virgin olive oil

- 2 tablespoons red wine vinegar

- 1 tablespoon Dijon mustard

- 1 clove garlic, minced

- Salt and pepper to taste

Instructions:

1. In a blender or food processor, combine sun-dried tomatoes, olive oil, red wine vinegar, Dijon mustard, garlic, salt, and pepper.

2. Blend until smooth.

Nutritional Information (per 2 tbsp serving):
Calories: 100, Protein: 1g, Fat: 9g, Carbohydrates: 2g

11. Spicy Peanut Sauce

Yields: *1 cup* **Prep time:** *5 minutes*

Ingredients:

- ¼ cup peanut butter
- 2 tablespoons soy sauce (or tamari for gluten-free)
- 2 tablespoons rice vinegar
- 1 tablespoon honey
- 1 teaspoon grated fresh ginger
- ½ teaspoon sriracha (or other hot sauce, adjust to taste)
- 2 tablespoons water (add more for desired consistency)

Instructions:

1. In a small bowl, whisk together all ingredients until smooth.

Nutritional Information (per 2 tbsp serving):

Calories: 120, Protein: 4g, Fat: 10g, Carbohydrates: 4g

12. Mango Salsa

Yields: *1 ½ cups* ***Prep time:*** *15 minutes*

Ingredients:

- 1 ripe mango, peeled and diced

- ½ cup chopped red onion

- ¼ cup chopped red bell pepper

- ¼ cup chopped fresh cilantro

- 2 tablespoons lime juice

- ¼ teaspoon salt

- Pinch of cayenne pepper (optional)

Instructions:

1. In a medium bowl, combine mango, red onion, bell pepper, cilantro, lime juice, salt, and cayenne pepper (if using).

Nutritional Information (per ¼ cup serving):
Calories: 40, Protein: 1g, Fat: 0g, Carbohydrates: 9g

13. Chimichurri Sauce

Yields: *1 cup* **Prep time:** *10 minutes*

Ingredients:

- 1 cup packed fresh parsley leaves
- ½ cup packed fresh cilantro leaves
- ¼ cup extra-virgin olive oil
- 2 tablespoons red wine vinegar
- 1 shallot, minced
- 2 cloves garlic, minced
- 1 teaspoon dried oregano
- ½ teaspoon red pepper flakes
- Salt and pepper to taste

Instructions:

1. In a food processor or blender, combine parsley, cilantro, olive oil, red wine vinegar, shallot, garlic, oregano, red pepper flakes, salt, and pepper.
2. Pulse until finely chopped, but not pureed.

Nutritional Information (per 2 tbsp serving):

Calories: 60, Protein: 1g, Fat: 6g, Carbohydrates: 1g

14. Creamy Dill Sauce for Salmon

Yields: *½ cup* ***Prep time:*** *5 minutes*

Ingredients:

- ½ cup plain Greek yogurt

- 2 tablespoons chopped fresh dill

- 1 tablespoon lemon juice

- Salt and pepper to taste

Instructions:

1. In a small bowl, stir together yogurt, dill, lemon juice, salt, and pepper.

Nutritional Information (per 2 tbsp serving):

Calories: 40, Protein: 4g, Fat: 2g, Carbohydrates: 1g

15. Lemon Garlic Butter Sauce for Seafood

Yields: *½ cup* ***Prep time:*** *5 minutes*

Ingredients:

- ¼ cup butter, melted

- 2 tablespoons lemon juice

- 2 cloves garlic, minced

- 1 tablespoon chopped fresh parsley

- Salt and pepper to taste

Instructions:

1. In a small bowl, whisk together melted butter, lemon juice, garlic, parsley, salt, and pepper.

Nutritional Information (per 2 tbsp serving):
Calories: 120, Protein: 0g, Fat: 14g, Carbohydrates: 0g

With these 15 flavorful dressings and sauces, you'll be well on your way to elevating your MIND diet meals to new heights of deliciousness. These recipes showcase the versatility and creativity that can be achieved with simple, wholesome ingredients, allowing you to enjoy a wide variety of flavors while adhering to the principles of healthy eating. So go ahead, drizzle, dip, and savor every bite of these culinary delights.

14-Day Meal Plan

"One cannot think well, love well, sleep well, if one has not dined well." Virginia Woolf's words resonate deeply with the essence of the MIND diet, emphasizing the connection between nourishment and overall well-being. Embarking on a new dietary pattern can be both exciting and overwhelming, but a well-structured meal plan can provide a roadmap for success.

This 14-day meal plan is designed to guide you through the initial stages of adopting the MIND diet, showcasing the delectable variety of recipes found within this book. Each day offers a harmonious balance of flavors, textures, and nutrients, ensuring you're enjoying the full spectrum of MIND-approved foods. The plan prioritizes simple preparations, readily available ingredients, and meals that can be easily adapted to your preferences and dietary needs.

Day 1

- **Breakfast:** Berry Blast Smoothie

- *(Nutritional Information: Calories: 250, Protein: 12g, Fat: 6g, Fiber: 8g)*

- **Lunch:** Mediterranean Chickpea Salad with Lemon-Tahini Dressing

- *(Nutritional Information (per serving): Calories: 450, Protein: 18g, Fat: 27g, Fiber: 14g)*

- **Dinner:** Lemon Herb Baked Salmon with Roasted Broccoli and Lemon Garlic

- *(Nutritional Information (combined per serving): Calories: 490, Protein: 34g, Fat: 28g, Fiber: 8g)*

Day 2

- **Breakfast:** Avocado Toast with Tomato and Feta

- *(Nutritional Information: Calories: 300, Protein: 10g, Fat: 18g, Fiber: 8g)*

- **Lunch:** Lemony Quinoa Salad with Asparagus and Dill

- *(Nutritional Information (per serving): Calories: 320, Protein: 10g, Fat: 15g, Fiber: 8g)*

- **Dinner:** Moroccan Chickpea and Sweet Potato Stew

- *(Nutritional Information (per serving): Calories: 450, Protein: 15g, Fat: 12g, Fiber: 18g)*

Day 3

- **Breakfast:** Savory Oatmeal with Spinach and Egg

- *(Nutritional Information: Calories: 280, Protein: 15g, Fat: 9g, Fiber: 7g)*

- **Lunch:** Kale Salad with Roasted Sweet Potato, Cranberries, and Pecans with Creamy Avocado Dressing

- *(Nutritional Information (combined per serving): Calories: 440, Protein: 9g, Fat: 25g, Fiber: 14g)*

- **Dinner:** Mediterranean Baked Cod with Tomatoes, Olives, and Capers

- *(Nutritional Information (per serving): Calories: 280, Protein: 25g, Fat: 12g)*

Day 4

- **Breakfast:** Berry Parfait with Granola and Nuts

- *(Nutritional Information: Calories: 350, Protein: 14g, Fat: 16g, Fiber: 8g)*

- **Lunch:** Black Bean and Corn Salad with Creamy Cilantro Lime Dressing

- *(Nutritional Information (combined per serving): Calories: 370, Protein: 14g, Fat: 19g, Fiber: 16g)*

- **Dinner:** Garlic Butter Shrimp Scampi with Zucchini Noodles

- *(Nutritional Information (per serving): Calories: 350, Protein: 35g, Fat: 15g)*

Day 5

- **Breakfast:** Tropical Green Smoothie

- *(Nutritional Information: Calories: 230, Protein: 4g, Fat: 3g, Fiber: 6g)*

- **Lunch:** Roasted Beetroot and Goat Cheese Salad with Walnuts & Honey Mustard Vinaigrette

- (Nutritional Information (combined per serving): Calories: 480, Protein: 12g, Fat: 37g, Fiber: 10g)

- **Dinner:** Spicy Tuna Salad with Avocado and Lime

- *(Nutritional Information (per serving without bread): Calories: 250, Protein: 25g, Fat: 12g)*

Day 6

- **Breakfast:** Banana Nut Oatmeal

- (Nutritional Information: Calories: 250, Protein: 8g, Fat: 7g, Fiber: 8g)

- **Lunch:** Asian Slaw with Peanut Ginger Dressing

- (Nutritional Information (per serving): Calories: 200, Protein: 5g, Fat: 12g, Fiber: 5g)

- **Dinner:** Pan-Seared Scallops with Brown Butter and Sage

- (Nutritional Information (per serving): Calories: 380, Protein: 25g, Fat: 25g)

Day 7

- **Breakfast:** Whole-Wheat Pancakes with Berries

- (Nutritional Information (per serving): Calories: 280, Protein: 10g, Fat: 10g, Fiber: 6g)

- **Lunch:** White Bean and Spinach Salad with Raspberry Vinaigrette

- (Nutritional Information (combined per serving): Calories: 380, Protein: 12g, Fat: 22g, Fiber: 13g)

- **Dinner:** Mediterranean Stuffed Eggplant

- *(Nutritional Information (per serving): Calories: 350, Protein: 12g, Fat: 18g, Fiber: 10g)*

Day 8

- **Breakfast:** Spinach and Feta Frittata

- *Nutritional Information (per serving): Calories: 200, Protein: 14g, Fat: 14g, Fiber: 1g*

- **Lunch:** Tomato and Cucumber Salad with Fresh Basil and Balsamic Vinaigrette

- (Nutritional Information (combined per serving): Calories: 270, Protein: 2g, Fat: 24g, Fiber: 4g)

- **Dinner:** Lentil and Vegetable Curry

- (Nutritional Information (per serving): Calories: 350, Protein: 15g, Fat: 8g, Fiber: 16g)

Day 9

- **Breakfast:** Berry Chia Seed Pudding

- *Nutritional Information: Calories: 250, Protein: 6g, Fat: 11g, Fiber: 15g*

- **Lunch:** Roasted Brussels Sprouts with Balsamic Glaze

- *(Nutritional Information (per serving): Calories: 180, Protein: 5g, Fat: 12g, Fiber: 8g)*

- **Dinner:** Vegetable Paella with Saffron and Artichoke Hearts

- *(Nutritional Information (per serving): Calories: 380, Protein: 10g, Fat: 12g, Fiber: 10g)*

Day 10

- **Breakfast:** Lemony Yogurt with Berries and Granola

- *Nutritional Information: Calories: 270, Protein: 12g, Fat: 8g, Fiber: 6g*

- **Lunch:** Roasted Carrots with Honey and Thyme

- *(Nutritional Information (per serving): Calories: 160, Protein: 2g, Fat: 9g, Fiber: 5g)*

- **Dinner:** Sweet Potato and Black Bean Burgers with Avocado Crema

- *(Nutritional Information (per serving): Calories: 400, Protein: 18g, Fat: 15g, Fiber: 12g)*

Day 11:

- **Breakfast:** Mediterranean Egg Scramble

- *(Nutritional Information: Calories: 250, Protein: 15g, Fat: 18g, Fiber: 2g)*

- **Lunch:** Grilled Zucchini and Summer Squash with Pesto

- *(Nutritional Information (per serving): Calories: 180, Protein: 3g, Fat: 15g, Fiber: 4g)*

- **Dinner:** Blackened Tilapia with Mango Salsa and Brown Rice

- *(Nutritional Information (combined per serving): Calories: 450, Protein: 28g, Fat: 12g, Fiber: 3g)*

Day 12:

- **Breakfast:** Tofu Scramble with Spinach and Tomatoes

- *(Nutritional Information: Calories: 280, Protein: 18g, Fat: 16g, Fiber: 5g)*

- **Lunch:** Roasted Asparagus with Lemon and Parmesan

- *(Nutritional Information (per serving): Calories: 120, Protein: 5g, Fat: 8g, Fiber: 3g)*

- **Dinner:** Salmon with Roasted Grapes and Balsamic Reduction

- *(Nutritional Information (per serving): Calories: 400, Protein: 30g, Fat: 25g)*

Day 13:

- **Breakfast:** Apple Cinnamon Baked Oatmeal

- *(Nutritional Information (per serving): Calories: 240, Protein: 8g, Fat: 8g, Fiber: 8g)*

- **Lunch:** Roasted Sweet Potato Wedges with Spicy Yogurt Dip

- *(Nutritional Information (per serving): Calories: 280, Protein: 8g, Fat: 12g, Fiber: 7g)*

- **Dinner:** Mediterranean Tuna Salad with White Beans and Artichoke Hearts on Whole-Wheat Bread

- *(Nutritional Information (per serving): Calories: 550, Protein: 38g, Fat: 28g, Fiber: 13g)*

Day 14:

- **Breakfast:** Smoked Salmon and Cream Cheese Egg Wraps

- *(Nutritional Information: Calories: 350, Protein: 20g, Fat: 25g, Fiber: 1g)*

- **Lunch:** Greek Salad with Olives and Feta and Sun-Dried Tomato Vinaigrette

- *(Nutritional Information (combined per serving): Calories: 350, Protein: 11g, Fat: 27g, Fiber: 7g)*

- **Dinner:** Baked Halibut with Tomato and Caper Relish

- *(Nutritional Information (per serving): Calories: 280, Protein: 25g, Fat: 12g)*

Beyond this 14-day plan, the possibilities are endless. Embrace the principles of the MIND diet, explore the diverse range of recipes in this book, and don't hesitate to experiment with new flavors and combinations. Remember, healthy eating is a journey, not a destination. By focusing on whole, unprocessed foods, you can nourish your body and mind while savoring the pleasures of the table.

Tips for Success:

- **Stay Hydrated:** Drink plenty of water throughout the day to maintain optimal health and energy levels.

- **Listen to Your Body:** Pay attention to your hunger and fullness cues. Eat when you're hungry, and stop when you're satisfied.

- **Get Creative in the Kitchen:** Don't be afraid to experiment with new recipes and flavor combinations. Cooking should be a joyful experience.

- **Share Meals with Loved Ones:** Eating with others can enhance the enjoyment of food and promote social connection.

- **Be Patient:** It takes time to establish new habits. Don't get discouraged if you slip up occasionally. Just get back on track and keep moving forward.

The MIND diet is not just a way of eating; it's a lifestyle that empowers you to take charge of your health and well-being. By embracing its principles, you can nourish your body and mind, reduce your risk of chronic diseases, and enhance your overall quality of life. So, let this 14-day meal plan be your starting point, and let the adventure begin!

Resources

"Knowledge is the food of the soul." This timeless quote by Plato highlights the importance of continuous learning and exploration, especially when it comes to our health and well-being. While this book provides a comprehensive guide to the MIND diet, it's just the beginning of your journey.

A wealth of resources awaits, ready to deepen your understanding, expand your culinary repertoire, and empower you to take charge of your brain health.

Organizations and Websites:

- **The Official MIND Diet Website:** This website offers a wealth of information on the MIND diet, including research findings, meal plans, shopping lists, and recipes. It's a great place to start your journey and stay up-to-date on the latest developments in MIND diet research.

- **National Institute on Aging:** This government agency provides reliable information on healthy aging, including nutrition, exercise, and cognitive health. Their website offers a variety of resources on the MIND diet and other dietary approaches to promote brain health.

- **Alzheimer's Association:** This leading voluntary health organization in Alzheimer's care, support, and research provides information and resources on the MIND diet as a potential strategy for reducing Alzheimer's risk.

Apps and Online Tools:

Several apps and online tools can help you track your MIND diet progress, find recipes, and create meal plans. These tools can be particularly helpful for those who are new to the diet or who need additional support in staying on track.

Local Resources:

Your local community may offer a variety of resources to support your MIND diet journey. Consider checking with your local library, senior center, or community health center for cooking classes, workshops, or support groups focused on the MIND diet.

Here are a few additional tips to help you make the most of the MIND diet:

- **Focus on whole, unprocessed foods:** Choose fruits, vegetables, whole grains, legumes, nuts, and seeds over processed foods, sugary drinks, and unhealthy fats.

- **Cook at home more often:** Cooking at home gives you more control over the ingredients in your food and allows you to experiment with different recipes.

- **Make gradual changes:** Don't try to overhaul your diet overnight. Start by incorporating more MIND-friendly foods into your meals and gradually reducing your intake of less healthy options.

- **Be mindful of portion sizes:** Even healthy foods can contribute to weight gain if you eat too much of them. Pay attention to your hunger and fullness cues and aim for moderate portions.

- **Enjoy the process:** The MIND diet is not about deprivation or restriction; it's about enjoying a variety of delicious and nutritious foods. Find recipes that you love and make healthy eating a pleasurable experience.

By utilizing these resources and incorporating these tips into your daily routine, you can successfully navigate the MIND diet and reap its benefits for your brain and overall health. Remember, knowledge is power, and the more you learn about the MIND diet, the more empowered you'll be to make informed choices that support your well-being.

References

Core Studies on the MIND Diet:

- Morris MC, Tangney CC, Wang Y, et al. MIND diet associated with reduced incidence of Alzheimer's disease. *Alzheimers Dement*. 2015 Sep;11(9):1007-14.

- Morris MC, Wang Y, Barnes LL, Bennett DA, Dawson-Hughes B, Booth SL. MIND diet slows cognitive decline with aging. *Alzheimers Dement*. 2015 Sep;11(9):1015-22.

- Li J, Wang Y, Barnes LL, Bennett DA, Schneider JA, Buchman AS, Wilson RS, Aggarwal NT, Morris MC. MIND and Mediterranean Diets Associated With Reduced Alzheimer's Disease Pathology. *Neurology*. 2023 Mar 14;100(11):e1225-e1235.

Research on the Mediterranean and DASH Diets:

- Sofi F, Abbate R, Gensini GF, Casini A, Macchi C, Abbate C, Fabiani L. Adherence to

Mediterranean diet and health status: meta-analysis. *BMJ*. 2008;337:a1344.

- Appel LJ, Moore TJ, Obarzanek E, et al. A clinical trial of the effects of dietary patterns on blood pressure. *N Engl J Med*. 1997;336(16):1117-24.

Studies on Specific Nutrients and Brain Health:

- Devore EE, Kang JH, Breteler MM, Grodstein F. Dietary intakes of berries and flavonoids in relation to cognitive decline. *Ann Neurol*. 2012 Jul;72(1):135-43.

- van de Rest O, Geleijnse JM, Kok FJ, van Staveren WA, Beek EM. Effect of fish oil on cognitive performance in older adults: a systematic review and meta-analysis of randomized clinical trials. *J Nutr Health Aging*. 2008;12(7):488-96.

- Clarke R, Smith AD, Jobst KA, Refsum H, Sutton L, Ueland PM. Folate, vitamin B12, and serum total homocysteine levels in confirmed Alzheimer disease. *Arch Neurol*. 1998;55(11):1449-55.

General Nutrition Resources for Seniors:

- National Institute on Aging: [invalid URL removed]

- Dietary Guidelines for Americans 2020-2025: https://www.dietaryguidelines.gov/

Additional Tips for Credibility:

- Cite all sources accurately and thoroughly.

- Include a reference list at the end of the book.

- Consider having a registered dietitian or nutritionist review your manuscript for accuracy and completeness.

- Highlight any personal anecdotes or testimonials from seniors who have successfully adopted the MIND diet.

By providing solid scientific backing for your claims and offering a wealth of additional resources, you can enhance the credibility of your cookbook and empower readers to make informed choices about their health.

Conversion Tables

Volume Conversions

Metric	U.S. Customary	Imperial
1 teaspoon (tsp)	1 teaspoon (tsp)	5 milliliters (ml)
1 tablespoon (tbsp)	1 tablespoon (tbsp)	15 milliliters (ml)
¼ cup	4 tablespoons (tbsp)	60 milliliters (ml)
⅓ cup	5 tablespoons (tbsp) + 1 teaspoon (tsp)	80 milliliters (ml)
½ cup	8 tablespoons (tbsp)	120 milliliters (ml)
⅔ cup	10 tablespoons (tbsp) + 2 teaspoons (tsp)	160 milliliters (ml)
¾ cup	12 tablespoons (tbsp)	180 milliliters (ml)
1 cup	16 tablespoons (tbsp)	240 milliliters (ml)

Weight Conversions

Metric	U.S. Customary	Imperial
1 ounce (oz)	28 grams (g)	28 grams (g)
4 ounces (oz)	¼ pound (lb)	113 grams (g)
8 ounces (oz)	½ pound (lb)	225 grams (g)
16 ounces (oz)	1 pound (lb)	450 grams (g)

Oven Temperature Conversions

Fahrenheit (°F)	Celsius (°C)	Description
200	95	Very low
250	120	Low
300	150	Moderate
350	175	Medium
375	190	Medium-high
400	200	High

Additional Tips:

- Invest in a kitchen scale for precise measurements, especially for baking.

- Use measuring cups and spoons designed for dry or liquid ingredients, respectively.

- When measuring sticky ingredients like honey or peanut butter, spray the measuring cup or spoon with cooking oil to prevent sticking.

- If a recipe calls for an ingredient you don't have, refer to a substitution chart or online resource for MIND diet-friendly alternatives.

This conversion table, coupled with the recipes and guidance throughout this book, equips you with the tools to confidently create delicious and nourishing MIND diet meals in your own kitchen.

TABLE OF CONTENT

INTRODUCTION

It's likely that if you're reading this, you either have gallbladder problems or have had your gallbladder removed. You're not by yourself! Gallbladder issues can be difficult, and feeling overwhelmed is common. Fortunately, you don't have to deal with this alone. I know what you're going through since I've worked with folks who have been in your situation. It can be quite taxing to deal with the pain, the anxiety, and the never-ending concern over whether your food will bring on more misery. But I can personally attest to the fact that altering your diet can have a profound impact. That's the reason this cookbook was made. I want to free you from the suffering that has been holding you back and empower you to take charge of your digestive health. You'll find tasty and healthful meals on these pages that are tailored to the needs of those without a gallbladder. You'll also receive helpful pointers and counsel on how to take care of your digestive system, stay away from triggers, and form wholesome routines.

This cookbook is for anyone who wants to:

- Learn how to navigate dietary changes after gallbladder removal

Discover easy and delicious recipes that cater to their new needs

- Improve their digestive health and nutrient absorption

- Find a supportive guide that understands what they're going through

Whether you're a beginner in the kitchen or a seasoned cook, this book is designed to be your trusted companion on the road to recovery. With simple language, easy-to-follow instructions, and vibrant photos, we'll take the mystery out of cooking without a gallbladder.

So, let's get started on this journey together! Every recipe, every tip, and every word in this book is here to help you feel better, inside and out. It's not just about cooking – it's about taking back control of your health and well-being. Let's do this!

CHAPTER 1: UNDERSTANDING THE ANATOMY OF THE GALLBLADDER

Where is the Gallbladder Located?

The gallbladder is a small organ located in the upper right side of your belly, just below your liver. It's about the size of a small pear.

What is the Structure of the Gallbladder?

The Gallbladder has Three Main Parts:

1. Fundus: The top part of the gallbladder, which is the widest section.

2. Body: The middle section where bile is stored.

3. Neck: The bottom part that connects the gallbladder to the bile duct.

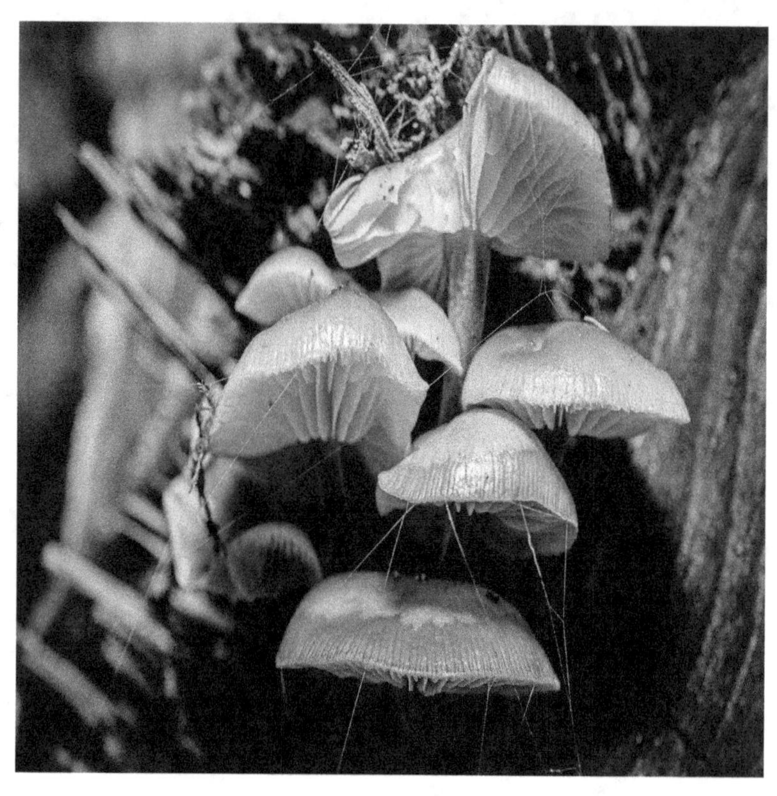

These three parts work together to help the gallbladder store and release bile, which helps with digestion.

Additionally, the gallbladder has three layers:

1. Mucosa: The inner layer that lines the inside of the gallbladder.

2. Muscle Layer: The middle layer that helps the gallbladder contract and release bile.

3. Serosa: The outer layer that covers the outside of the gallbladder.

These layers and parts work together to keep the gallbladder functioning properly.

Symptoms and Causes

Gallbladder Problems: Know the Symptoms

If your gallbladder isn't working properly, you may experience:

1. Abdominal Pain: Pain in the upper right side of your belly, which can be sharp or dull.

2. Nausea and Vomiting: Feeling queasy or sick to your stomach, which can lead to vomiting.

3. Fever: A high temperature, usually above 100.4°F(38°C).

4. Chills: Feeling cold and having shakes or shivers.

5. Yellowing of the Skin and Eyes (Jaundice): A yellow tint to your skin and the whites of your eyes.

6. Tea-Colored Urine: Urine that's darker than usual, like tea.

7. Shaking or Shaking Feelings: Feeling weak or trembly.

8. Loss of Appetite: Not feeling like eating or drinking.

9. Bloating and Gas: Feeling full or swollen in your belly.

10. Diarrhea: Loose, watery stools or frequent bowel movements.

If you're experiencing any of these symptoms, it's important to see a doctor to find out what's going on and get the right treatment.

Causes

What Causes Gallbladder Problems?

Several things can lead to gallbladder problems, including:

- Gallstones: Small, hard deposits that form in the gallbladder, often made of cholesterol or bilirubin.

- Blockage: When a gallstone or other material blocks the bile ducts, preventing bile from flowing.

- Inflammation: When the gallbladder becomes swollen and irritated, often due to infection.

- Genetics: A family history of gallbladder problems can increase your risk.

- Hormonal Changes: Changes in hormone levels during pregnancy, menopause, or birth control pill use.

- Obesity: Being overweight or obese can increase the risk of gallbladder problems.

- Diabetes: Having diabetes can increase the risk of gallbladder problems.

- Rapid Weight Loss: Losing weight too quickly can increase the risk of gallbladder problems.

- Age: Risk increases after age 60.

- Gender: Women are more likely to develop gallbladder problems than men.

These factors can increase the likelihood of gallbladder problems, but it's important to note that sometimes the cause may not be known.

Diagnoses and Tests

Diagnosing Gallbladder Problems

When you visit your healthcare professional, they will start by asking about your medical history and symptoms. They will also check your vital signs, such as heart rate, blood pressure, and body temperature, to see if you have a fever.

Next, they will perform a physical exam to check for signs of jaundice (yellowing of the skin and eyes) and abdominal swelling. They will also press on your abdominal area to feel your gallbladder. If it's inflamed, they may be able to feel it. This can help them determine if you have acute inflammation (usually caused by gallstones) or chronic inflammation (which could be a sign of cancer).

Your physician may also prescribe further tests, such as:

- Blood tests to detect evidence of infection or inflammation.

- Imaging tests like ultrasound, CT scans, or MRI to visualize your gallbladder and bile ducts

These tests will help your healthcare professional determine the cause of your symptoms and develop an appropriate treatment plan.

Remember that your healthcare professional is there to help you. Don't hesitate to ask questions or share your concerns. With the right diagnosis and treatment, you can feel better soon!

Tests for Gallbladder Problems

Your healthcare professional may order one or more of the following tests to diagnose gallbladder problems:

- Complete Blood Count (CBC): This blood test checks for signs of infection or inflammation by measuring white blood cell levels.

- Liver Function Tests: These blood tests help detect bile duct obstructions by measuring liver enzymes.

- Pancreatic Function Tests: These blood tests diagnose pancreatic duct blockages by measuring pancreatic enzymes.

- Abdominal Ultrasound: This non-invasive imaging test uses sound waves to visualize the gallbladder, bile ducts, and surrounding organs, detecting inflammation, obstructions, or growths.

- HIDA Scan (Cholescintigraphy): This imaging test evaluates gallbladder function and bile flow through the bile ducts, helping diagnose blockages or inflammation.

- Endoscopic Retrograde Cholangiopancreatography (ERCP): This test combines endoscopy and X-ray technology to visualize the bile ducts and pancreas. A flexible tube with a camera and light is inserted through your mouth to detect blockages or stones, which can be removed during the procedure.

- Endoscopic Ultrasound (EUS): This test uses ultrasound technology and endoscopy to visualize the gallbladder, bile ducts, pancreas, and liver. A special endoscope with ultrasound capabilities is inserted through your mouth to detect abnormalities, which may require further testing or procedures.

These tests help your healthcare professional diagnose and treat gallbladder problems effectively.

Surgical Options for Gallbladder Problems

If tests show gallstones, inflammation, or other serious gallbladder issues, surgery might be the best option. The most common surgical procedure is a cholecystectomy, which means removing the gallbladder.

This can be accomplished in two ways:

Laparoscopic surgery: A minimally invasive procedure using small incisions and a camera to guide the surgeon.

- Open surgery: A more traditional approach, used when necessary, which involves a larger incision.

Surgery is usually considered when:

- Symptoms persist or recur

- Complications arise

- Imaging tests reveal significant findings

Removing the gallbladder can provide relief from symptoms and prevent future complications. Your healthcare professional will discuss the best course of action for your specific situation.

CHAPTER 2:

GALLBLADDER REMOVAL SURGERY

Gallbladder removal surgery, also known as cholecystectomy, takes out a diseased gallbladder. This operation is often done laparoscopically, which means:

- Small incisions (cuts) are made in your abdomen

- A lighted tube (scope) and surgical equipment are inserted

- Air is used to inflate your stomach, allowing the surgeon to see your organs clearly

- With time, the incisional scars will disappear.

In some cases, open surgery is the better option. Your doctor may decide on open surgery beforehand or switch to it during a laparoscopic operation. Open surgery involves:

- A larger incision in your upper abdomen

- A hospital stay of 2-4 days

- A recovery time of 4-6 weeks before returning to your normal routine

Remember, your doctor will discuss the best approach for your specific situation.

Preparing for Surgery: A Checklist

1. Arrange a ride home:

Make sure someone can drive you home after surgery, as anesthesia and pain medication can impair your ability to drive or travel alone.

2. Understand the procedure:

Ask your doctor to explain the surgery, including benefits, risks, and options, so you know what to expect.

3. A Blood thinners:

If you take blood thinners, consult your doctor about stopping them before surgery, as they can increase bleeding risks. Follow their instructions carefully.

4. Medications and supplements:

Inform your doctor about all medications, vitamins, and natural health products you take, as some may cause complications during surgery. Your doctor will advise you on which ones to stop taking before surgery.

5. Advance care plan: Ensure your doctor and hospital have a copy of your advance care plan, which outlines your healthcare preferences.

If you don't have one, consider creating one before surgery.

By following these steps, you'll be well-prepared for your surgery and can focus on a smooth recovery.

The Day of Surgery: What to Expect

1. Fasting instructions: Follow the guidelines for when to stop eating and drinking. Your surgery might be canceled if you don't. Medications: If your doctor told you to take your medications on the day of surgery, take them with a small sip of water.

3. Personal hygiene:

  - Take a bath or shower to prepare for surgery

  - Avoid using lotions, perfumes, deodorants, or nail polish

4. Shaving: Don't shave the area where the surgery will take place

5. Jewelry and piercings: Remove all jewelry and piercings

6. Contact lenses: Take out your contact lenses

By following these steps, you'll be well-prepared for your surgery. Remember to ask your doctor if you have any questions or concerns!

At the Hospital or Surgery Center:

1. Bring your photo ID: Make sure to bring a valid government-issued ID to the hospital or surgery center.

2. Surgical site marking: To ensure accuracy, the surgical site will be marked to avoid any mistakes.

3. Anesthesia care: Your anesthesiologist will ensure your comfort and safety throughout the procedure. Throughout the procedure, you will be unconscious.

4. Surgery duration: The operation typically takes 1 to 2 hours to complete.

Remember, your healthcare team is dedicated to providing you with quality care and a smooth experience. If you have any questions or issues, please don't hesitate to ask!

When to Contact Your Doctor

- Questions or concerns: If you have any questions or concerns about your surgery, don't hesitate to reach out to your doctor.

- Preparation uncertainty: If you're unsure about how to prepare for surgery, contact your doctor for guidance.

- Illness before surgery: If you develop a fever, flu, cold, or any other illness before surgery, contact your doctor immediately.

- Change of heart or schedule: If you want to reschedule or cancel your surgery, or if you've changed your mind about the procedure, contact your doctor as soon as possible.

Remember, your doctor is there to support you throughout the process. Don't hesitate to reach out if you need anything!

Your recovery after surgery

After Your Surgery

- Weakness and fatigue: You'll likely feel weak and tired for several days after returning home from surgery.

- Bloating and discomfort: Your stomach may feel swollen, and you may experience shoulder soreness (if you had laparoscopic surgery) due to the air used to inflate your stomach.

- Digestive changes: You may experience gas, burping, or diarrhea (which usually resolves within 2-4 weeks).

- Recovery time:

Laparoscopic surgery: Most people return to work or normal activities within 1-2 weeks, but recovery time varies depending on your job.

Open surgery: It usually takes 4-6 weeks to return to your usual routine.

Remember, everyone's recovery is different. Be patient, and follow your doctor's instructions to ensure a smooth recovery.

Home care

Activity Guidelines After Surgery

- Rest and sleep: Listen to your body and rest when you're tired. Adequate sleep aids in recovery.

- Walking: Aim to walk daily, gradually increasing your distance each day. Walking helps prevent blood clots and pneumonia.

- Lifting restrictions: Avoid carrying heavy objects (like children, heavy bags, or vacuum cleaners) for 2-4 weeks.

- Intense activities: Consult your doctor before resuming activities like bicycling, running, weightlifting, or aerobics.

- Driving: Ask your doctor when it's safe to drive again.

- Return to work/routine:

Laparoscopic surgery: Usually 1-2 weeks, but may vary.

Open surgery: Typically 4-6 weeks.

Sexual activity: Consult your doctor to determine when it's safe to resume sexual activity.

Remember, everyone's recovery pace is different. Follow your doctor's guidance to ensure a smooth and safe recovery.

Diet and Medicines After Surgery

Diet:

Start with small portions: Eat modest amounts when you're hungry. We'll discuss diet details, including what to eat and avoid, in the next chapter.

Medicines:

Resume medications: Your doctor will advise when to restart your medications.

Blood thinners: If you stopped taking aspirin or other blood thinners, consult your doctor about when to resume.

Medication safety:

Read and follow label instructions carefully.

Take pain medicine exactly as prescribed by your doctor.

If you don't have a prescription for pain medication, consult your doctor about over-the-counter options.

Remember, always follow your doctor's guidance on diet and medication to ensure a safe and smooth recovery.

Pain Medication and Wound Care

Pain Medication:

- Use pain medication only as prescribed: Avoid taking excessive pain medication, as it can be harmful. Many pain relievers contain acetaminophen (Tylenol), which can be dangerous in high doses.

- Managing nausea: Take medication after meals (unless advised otherwise). Ask your doctor for alternative pain medication if nausea persists.

Antibiotics:

- Complete the full course: Take antibiotics exactly as directed and finish the entire prescription, even if you feel better before completing the course.

Wound Care:

- Keep the incision dry: Leave tape strips on for a week or until they fall off.

- Showering: Showering is allowed 24-48 hours after surgery, with doctor's approval. Gently pat the incision dry.

- Bathing: Avoid bathing for the first two weeks or until your doctor says it's safe.

- Staples: Keep staples dry until your doctor removes them (usually 7-10 days).

- Dressings: Keep the area clean and dry. If fluid seeps or the incision rubs against clothing, cover it with a gauze bandage and change daily.

- Remember, always follow your doctor's instructions for pain management and wound care to ensure a safe and smooth recovery.

Ice

Using Ice for Recovery

- Apply ice or a cold compress to your tummy for 10-20 minutes

- Repeat every 1-2 hours to reduce swelling and soreness

- Put a little cloth between the ice and your skin.

Follow-up Care

-Attend all scheduled appointments

- Contact your doctor or nurse advice line (811 in most provinces and territories) if you have any concerns.

- Keep track of your test results and meds.

Remember, follow-up care is crucial for your recovery and safety. By staying connected with your healthcare team and monitoring your progress, you can ensure a smooth and successful recovery.

When to Call for Help

Emergency Situations

- Call 911 immediately if you:

Lose consciousness or pass out

Feel short of breath

Urgent Concerns

Contact your doctor or nurse right away if you:

Have severe stomach pain or inability to drink water

Experience persistent pain despite taking pain medication

Are unable to pass stools or gas

Show signs of infection (increased pain, swelling, warmth, redness, or pus)

Notice loose stitches or an open incision

Experience bleeding through the bandage covering your incision

Potential Complications

Watch for signs of deep vein thrombosis (DVT):

Pain in the calf, back of knee, thigh, or groin

Redness and swelling in the groin or leg.

General Guidance

Monitor your health closely and call your doctor or nurse advice line if you have any concerns or questions.

Remember, it's always better to err on the side of caution and seek medical attention if you're unsure about your symptoms or condition.

CHAPTER 3:

DIET GUIDE - FOODS TO INCLUDE AND AVOID

Diet Guide After Gallbladder Removal

Introduction

• Without a gallbladder, bile flows freely into the small intestine, reducing its ability to break down food.

• Dietary modifications may be necessary to compensate, but these adjustments may only be temporary.

Foods to Avoid

• Fatty, oily, processed, and sugary foods

• Foods high in eggs, animal protein, and saturated fat

• Low vegetable intake

Symptoms and Concerns

• Consuming these foods may lead to:

Gas

Bloating

Diarrhea

• These symptoms are not major health concerns but can be uncomfortable.

Next Steps

- Gradually introduce some of these foods back into your diet in the months following surgery.

- Monitor your body's reaction and adjust your diet accordingly.

Remember, everyone's digestive system is unique, so it's essential to listen to your body and make adjustments as needed.

Foods to Avoid: Meats and Dairy

Fatty Meats

- Processed or high-fat meats can cause digestive issues after gallbladder removal

Examples:

Steak

Beef

Pork

Bacon

Lunch meats (bologna, salami)

Sausage

Lamb

Dairy Products

• Can be difficult to digest after gallbladder removal

• Avoid or restrict:

Whole milk

Full-fat yogurt

Full-fat cheese

Butter

Lard

Sour cream

Ice cream

Whipped cream

Cream-based sauces and gravies

Alternatives

If you can't give up dairy, consider:

Fat-free yogurt

Low-fat cheese

Non-dairy substitutes (e.g., almond milk)

Foods to Avoid: Processed Foods

Highly processed foods:

High in added fat and sugar

Difficult to digest

Low in nutrients

Examples to avoid:

Pie

Cake

Cookies

Cinnamon rolls

Sugary cereals

White or processed bread

Foods cooked in vegetable or partly hydrogenated oils

Foods to Include

While some foods should be avoided, there are many nutritious options to choose from

Focus on whole, unprocessed foods:

Vegetables

Fruits

Whole grains

Lean proteins

Healthy fats

Note: It's important to consult with a healthcare professional or a registered dietitian for personalized dietary advice after gallbladder removal.

High-Fiber Foods

Fiber can aid digestion in the absence of concentrated bile

Gradually increase fiber intake to avoid gas and discomfort after surgery

Good Sources of Fiber and Other Nutrients

- Legumes:

Beans

Lentils

Peas

- Whole grains:

Skinned potatoes

Oatmeal

Barley

Whole grain bread, pasta, rice, and cereal

- Nuts and seeds:

Raw nuts (almonds, walnuts, cashews)

Raw seeds (hemp, chia, poppy)

Sprouted grains, nuts, and seeds

Fresh fruits and vegetables:

Rich in nutrients and vitamins

Aim to include a variety of nutrient-dense options

Remember to consult with your healthcare provider or a registered dietitian for personalized dietary advice after gallbladder removal.

Healing Foods

- High in antioxidants, fiber, vitamin C, and phytonutrients to support healing:

Brussels sprouts

Cauliflower

Broccoli

Kale

Legumes (peas, lentils, beans)

Cabbage

Tomatoes

Spinach

Citrus fruits (oranges, limes)

Avocados

Berries (blueberries, blackberries, raspberries)

Lean Protein Sources

• Choose lean meats or plant-based options:

Chicken breast

Turkey

Salmon

Trout

Herring

Whitefish

Lentils

Tofu

Remember, a balanced diet with a variety of whole foods can help support your recovery after gallbladder removal surgery.

Healthy Fats and Low-Fat Options

- Use healthy fats like avocado oil, olive oil, and coconut oil instead of vegetable oil

- Limit oil usage overall

- Replace high-fat foods with low-fat alternatives:

Mayonnaise

Milk

Yogurt

Sour cream or ice cream

Additional Diet Tips

- Make small dietary changes to aid in smooth recovery

- Consider the following:

Delay introducing solid foods after surgery

Gradually reintroduce solid foods to avoid stomach issues

Eat smaller, frequent meals throughout the day

Avoid eating too much at once to prevent gas and bloating

Aim for 5-6 small meals per day, spaced a few hours apart

Snack on nutrient-dense, low-fat, high-protein snacks between meals.

- Limit fat intake to 3 grams per meal

- Substitute ingredients in recipes:

Use applesauce instead of butter in baking

Replace eggs with flaxseed and water mixture

- Consider adopting a vegetarian diet:

Meat and dairy, especially full-fat versions, can be harder to digest without a gallbladder

- Maintain physical fitness:

Regular exercise and a healthy weight can improve digestion

Important Note

Before trying any new recipes, consult with your doctor to ensure they are suitable for your individual needs.

CHAPTER 4:

BREAKFAST

Start the day with a delicious and nutritious breakfast. Breakfast is the most important meal of the day, and it's especially crucial for maintaining good digestive health. In this chapter, we'll explore a variety of breakfast recipes that are not only delicious but also packed with nutrients to help soothe and support your digestive system. From filling quinoa porridge to light and fluffy pancakes, there's something for everyone to enjoy. Let's dive in and make every morning a delight!

Quinoa Porridge with Cinnamon and Apples

Description: A warm, comforting, and nutritious breakfast porridge that combines the goodness of quinoa with the sweet, aromatic flavors of cinnamon and apples. Perfect for a gallbladder-friendly meal to start your day.

Cooking Time: 20 minutes

Prep Time: 10 minutes

Servings: 4

Ingredients:

1 cup quinoa, rinsed

2 cups water

1 cup almond milk (or the dairy-free milk of your choice)

2 apples, peeled, cored, and diced

1 tsp ground cinnamon

2 tbsp maple syrup or honey

1/4 tsp salt

1/4 cup chopped walnuts (optional)

Fresh mint leaves for garnish (optional)

Nutritional Information (per serving)

Calories: 230

Protein: 6g

Carbohydrates: 40g

Dietary Fiber: 5g

Sugars: 12g

Fat: 6g

Saturated Fat: 0.5g

Sodium: 120mg

Preparation Steps

1. Cook the Quinoa:

In a medium saucepan, mix the quinoa and water.

Bring to a boil over medium-high heat.

Reduce the heat to low, cover, and cook for about 15 minutes, or until the quinoa is cooked and the water is absorbed.

2. Prepare the Apple Mixture:

In a separate small saucepan, combine diced apples, almond milk, cinnamon, maple syrup or honey, and salt.

Cook over medium heat until apples are tender, about 5 minutes.

3. Combine and Thicken:

Stir the apple mixture into the cooked quinoa.

Continue to cook for an additional 2-3 minutes, stirring frequently until the porridge thickens to your desired consistency.

4. Serve and Enjoy:

Serve warm, topped with chopped walnuts and fresh mint leaves if desired.

Oatmeal with Berries and Almonds

Description: A nutritious and delicious breakfast option that combines oats with crunchy almonds, fresh berries, and antioxidant-rich fruits.

Cooking Time: 10 minutes

Prep Time: 5 minutes

Servings: 2

Ingredients:

1 cup rolled oats

2 cups water or almond milk

1/2 tsp vanilla extract

1/4 tsp ground cinnamon

1 cup mixed berries (including blueberries, strawberries, and raspberries)

2 tbsp sliced almonds

1 tbsp chia seeds (optional)

1-2 tsp honey or maple syrup (optional)

Fresh mint leaves for garnish (optional)

Nutritional Information (per serving)

Calories: 290

Protein: 8g

Carbohydrates: 50g

Dietary Fiber: 8g

Sugars: 10g

Fat: 9g

Saturated Fat: 0.5g

Sodium: 1mg

Preparation Steps

1. Cook the Oats:

In a medium saucepan, heat the water or almond milk until it boils.

Stir in the rolled oats, reduce the heat to medium, and cook for 5 minutes, stirring occasionally.

2. Add Flavorings:

Stir in the vanilla extract and ground cinnamon until thoroughly combined.

3. Achieve Desired Consistency:

Continue to cook until the oats reach your desired consistency, about 2-3 more minutes.

4. Assemble and Serve:

Divide the oatmeal into two bowls.

Garnish each bowl with mixed berries, sliced almonds, and chia seeds.

Drizzle with honey or maple syrup if desired.

Garnish with fresh mint leaves.

Avocado and Egg Wrap

Description: A quick and delicious breakfast wrap that combines creamy avocado with protein-packed eggs, perfect for a healthy, on-the-go meal that gently soothes the digestive system.

Cooking Time: 5 minutes

Prep Time: 5 minutes

Servings: 1

Ingredients:

1 whole wheat tortilla

1 ripe avocado, peeled and pitted

2 large eggs

1 tbsp olive oil

Salt and pepper to taste

1/4 cup cherry tomatoes, halved

1 tbsp chopped fresh cilantro

Lime wedge (optional)

Nutritional Information (per serving):

Calories: 350

Protein: 14g

Carbohydrates: 28g

Dietary Fiber: 10g

Sugars: 3g

Fat: 22g

Saturated Fat: 4g

Sodium: 290 mg

Preparation Steps

1. Mash the Avocado:

In a small bowl, use a fork to mash the avocado until smooth.

Season with salt and pepper to taste.

Cook the Eggs:

In a nonstick skillet, heat the olive oil on medium heat.

Crack the eggs into the skillet and cook to your desired doneness level (sunny side up, over easy, or scrambled).

Warm the Tortilla:

Warm the tortilla in a dry skillet or microwave for 30 seconds until pliable.

Assemble the Wrap:

Spread the mashed avocado on the tortilla.

Place cooked eggs on top of the avocado.

Add the halved cherry tomatoes and sprinkle with chopped cilantro.

Fold and Serve:

Fold the tortilla sides over the filling, then roll it up from the bottom.

Serve with a lime wedge if desired.

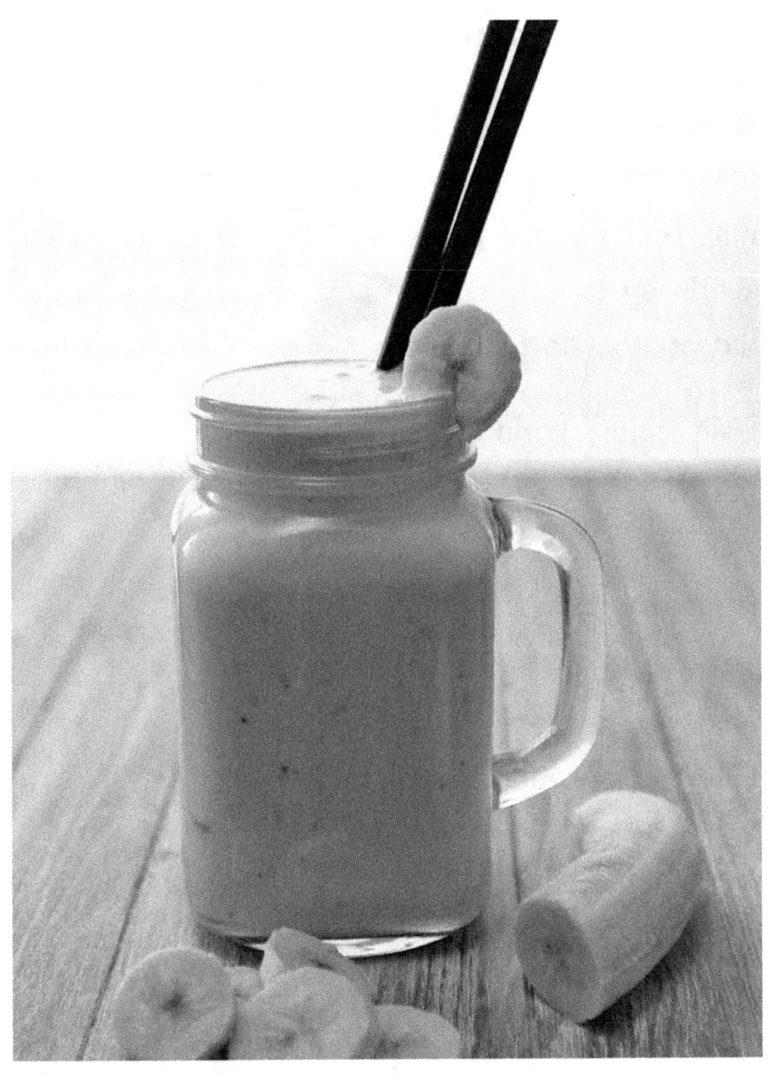

Banana Nut Smoothie

Description: A creamy and nutritious smoothie that's perfect for breakfast or a snack. With bananas, nuts, and a hint of cinnamon, it's both delicious and gentle on the digestive system, making it ideal for those without a gallbladder.

Prep Time: 5 minutes

Servings: 2

Ingredients:

2 ripe bananas

1 cup unsweetened almond milk

1/2 cup Greek yogurt (or dairy-free alternative)

2 tbsp almond butter

1 tbsp chia seeds

1/2 tsp ground cinnamon

1 tsp honey or maple syrup (optional)

Ice cubes (optional)

Nutritional Information (per serving):

Calories: 250

Protein: 7g

Carbohydrates: 38g

Dietary Fiber: 7g

Sugars: 18g

Fat: 10g

Saturated Fat: 1g

Sodium: 90

Preparation Steps

1. Blend the Ingredients:

In a blender, combine the bananas, almond milk, Greek yogurt, almond butter, chia seeds, and ground cinnamon.

Blend until smooth and creamy.

2. Add Sweetness (Optional):

Add honey or maple syrup if you desire a sweeter smoothie.

Blend until well combined.

3. Add Ice (Optional):

Add ice cubes if you prefer a colder, thicker smoothie.

Blend until smooth and creamy.

4. Serve and Enjoy:

Pour the smoothie into two glasses.

Serve immediately and enjoy!

Blueberry Banana Pancakes

Description: Fluffy pancakes packed with banana natural sweetness and blueberry antioxidant power, making them a healthy and delicious breakfast choice for a gallbladder-friendly diet.

Cooking Time: 15 minutes

Prep Time: 10 minutes

Servings: 4

Ingredients:

1 cup whole wheat flour

1 tbsp baking powder

1/4 tsp salt

1 cup almond milk

1 large ripe banana, mashed

1 tbsp maple syrup

1 tsp vanilla extract

1 cup fresh or frozen blueberries

Cooking spray or a small amount of oil for the pan

Nutritional Information (per serving):

Calories: 210

Protein: 5g

Carbohydrates: 40g

Dietary Fiber: 6g

Sugars: 12g

Fat: 3g

Saturated Fat: 0.5g

Sodium: 250mg

Preparation Steps:

1. Whisk Dry Ingredients:

In a large mixing bowl, whisk together whole wheat flour, baking powder, and salt.

2. Combine Wet Ingredients:

In a separate bowl, combine almond milk, mashed banana, maple syrup, and vanilla extract. Mix well.

3. Combine Wet and Dry Ingredients:

Pour the wet ingredients into the dry ingredients and whisk until they incorporate. Do not overmix.

4. Fold in Blueberries:

Gently fold in the blueberries.

Cook Pancakes:

Heat a non-stick skillet or griddle over medium heat
and lightly coat with cooking spray or oil.

Pour 1/4 cup batter into the skillet per pancake.
Cook until bubbles appear on the surface, then flip
and cook until golden brown on the opposite side.

5. Serve and Enjoy:

Serve warm, topped with additional blueberries and
maple syrup drizzle if desired.

Veggie Omelette with Spinach

Description: A nutrient-packed veggie omelet featuring fresh spinach, vibrant vegetables, and protein-rich eggs, perfect for a delicious and satisfying breakfast that will keep you energized all morning long.

Cooking Time: 10 minutes

Prep Time: 10 minutes

Servings: 2

Ingredients:

2 large eggs

1/4 cup almond milk

1/4 cup sliced mushrooms

1/2 cup fresh spinach leaves

1/4 cup diced bell peppers

1 tbsp olive oil

Salt and pepper to taste

Fresh parsley for garnish (optional)

Nutritional Information (per serving):

Calories: 220

Total Fat: 14g

Saturated Fat: 4g

Sodium: 200mg

Total Carbohydrates: 6g

Dietary Fiber: 2g

Sugars: 3g

Protein: 16g

Preparation Steps

Whisk Egg Mixture:

In a medium mixing basin, whisk together the eggs and milk until thoroughly blended.

Season with salt and pepper to taste.

Sauté Vegetables:

Heat the olive oil or butter in a nonstick skillet over medium heat.

Add the chopped red onion and bell pepper to the skillet. Sauté for 2-3 minutes, or until the vegetables begin to soften.

Add Tomatoes and Spinach:

Add the cherry tomatoes and chopped spinach to the skillet. Cook for another 2 minutes, stirring occasionally, until the spinach is wilted.

Pour Egg Mixture:

Pour the egg mixture over the vegetables in the skillet, tilting the pan to spread it evenly.

Let it cook undisturbed for 1-2 minutes, or until the edges start to set.

Add Cheese (Optional):

If using cheese, sprinkle it over the omelet at this stage.

Cook and Fold:

Using a spatula, gently lift the edges of the omelet and tilt the pan to allow the uncooked eggs to flow to the edges.

Continue to cook for another 2-3 minutes, or until the eggs are fully set and the cheese is melted.

Serve and Enjoy:

Carefully fold the omelet in half and transfer to a plate.

Garnish with fresh herbs and serve immediately.

Chia Seed Pudding with Fresh Fruit

Description: A versatile and nutrient-dense breakfast or snack option that's easy to prepare, high in fiber, and pairs wonderfully with fresh fruit for a refreshing and gallbladder-friendly meal.

Prep Time: 10 minutes

Servings: 2

Ingredients:

1/4 cup chia seeds

1 cup unsweetened almond milk

1 tbsp honey or maple syrup

1/2 tsp vanilla extract

Fresh fruit for topping (such as strawberries, kiwi, or mango)

Mint leaves for garnish (optional)

Nutritional Information (per serving):

Calories: 180

Protein: 4g

Carbohydrates: 22g

Dietary Fiber: 8g

Sugars: 12g

Fat: 8g

Saturated Fat: 0.5g

Sodium: 60mg

Preparation Steps

1. Whisk Chia Seed Mixture:

In a medium bowl, whisk together chia seeds, almond milk, honey or maple syrup, and vanilla extract until well combined.

2. Refrigerate and Thicken:

Cover the bowl and refrigerate for at least 4 hours or overnight, allowing the chia seeds to swell and the mixture to thicken.

3. Serve and Top:

Stir the pudding before serving, then divide it into two bowls.

Top with fresh fruit and garnish with mint leaves if desired.

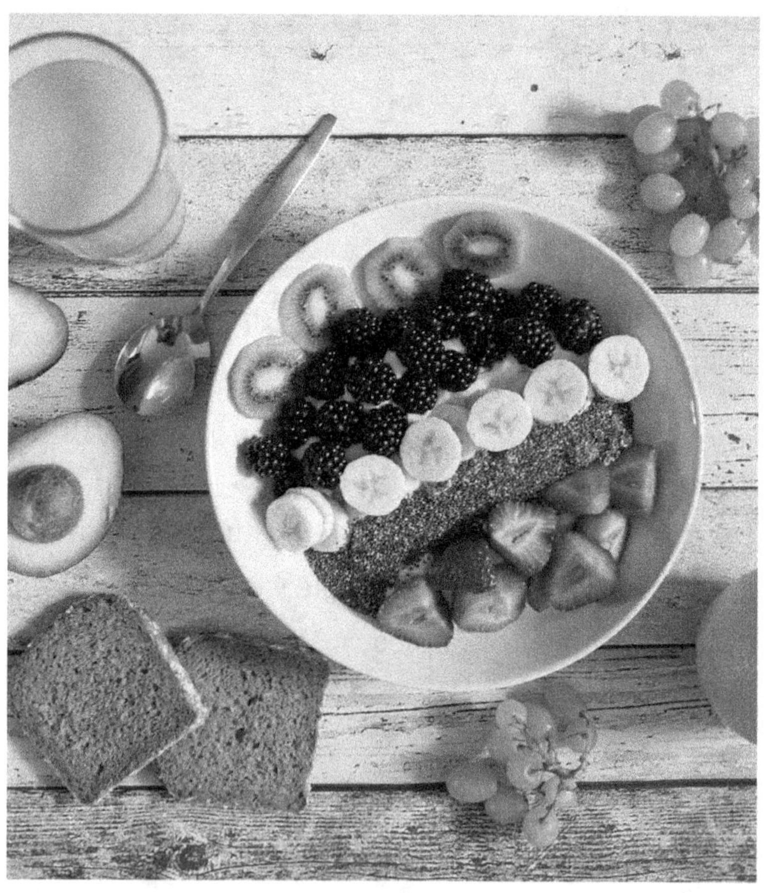

Burrito Bowl

Description: A deconstructed breakfast burrito bowl packed with vegetables, protein, and healthy fats, making it a delicious and gallbladder-friendly option to kick-start your day.

Cooking Time: 10 minutes

Prep Time: 10 minutes

Servings: 2

Ingredients:

Nutritional Information (per serving):

Calories: 400

Protein: 18g

Carbohydrates: 45g

Dietary Fiber: 12g

Sugars: 6g

Fat: 19g

Saturated Fat: 3g

Sodium: 350mg

Preparation Steps:

1. Scramble Eggs:

Heat the olive oil in a nonstick skillet over medium heat.

Crack the eggs into the skillet and scramble until fully done.

Season with salt and pepper.

2. Assemble Bowls:

Divide the cooked quinoa between two bowls.

Top each bowl with scrambled eggs, black beans, diced avocado, cherry tomatoes, and red onion.

3. Add Salsa and Cilantro:

Add a spoonful of salsa to each bowl and sprinkle with chopped cilantro.

4. Serve and Enjoy:

Optional: serve with lime wedges on the side.

Spinach and Feta Quiche

Description: A light and flavorful quiche perfect for breakfast or brunch, made with a whole wheat crust, fresh spinach, and tangy feta cheese.

Cooking Time: 35 minutes

Prep Time: 15 minutes

Servings: 6

Ingredients:

1 whole wheat pie crust

1 tbsp olive oil

1 small onion, diced

3 cups fresh spinach, chopped

4 large eggs

1 cup unsweetened almond milk

1/2 cup crumbled feta cheese

1/4 tsp salt

1/4 tsp ground black pepper

1/4 tsp ground nutmeg (optional)

Nutritional Information (per serving):

Calories: 220

Protein: 10g

Carbohydrates: 20g

Dietary Fiber: 3g

Sugars: 2g

Fat: 12g

Saturated Fat: 4g

Sodium: 360mg

Preparation Steps

1. Preheat the Oven and Prepare the Crust:

Preheat the oven to 375°F (190°C).

Put the pie crust in a 9-inch pie dish and set aside.

2. Sauté Onion and Spinach:

In a medium-size skillet, heat the olive oil.

Sauté the diced onion until transparent, about 5 minutes.

 Cook the chopped spinach in the skillet until wilted, about 2-3 minutes.

Remove from heat and allow it to cool slightly.

3. Prepare Egg Mixture:

In a large bowl, whisk together the eggs, almond milk, salt, pepper, and nutmeg (if using).

4. Assemble Quiche:

Spread the spinach-onion mixture evenly over the pie crust.

Sprinkle crumbled feta cheese on top.

Pour the egg mixture over the spinach and feta into the pie crust.

5. Bake and Cool:

Bake in the preheated oven for 30-35 minutes, or until the quiche is set and lightly golden on top.

Let cool before slicing and serving.

CHAPTER 5:

SNACKS AND APPETIZERS

Welcome to our next chapter! Here, we'll explore delicious and healthy snack options that are gentle on our digestive system. From creamy dips to crunchy treats, these recipes will keep you full and energized throughout the day.

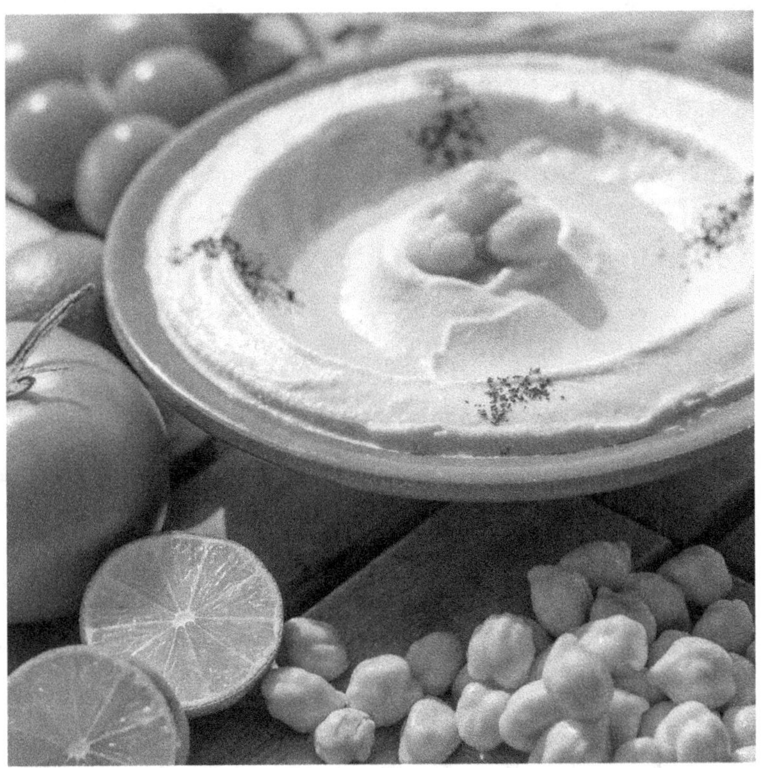

Hummus and Veggie Sticks

This classic snack is easy to make and packed with nutrients. It's high in fiber and protein, making it perfect for a balanced diet that's gentle on the gallbladder.

Prep Time: 10 minutes

Servings: 4

Ingredients:

1 cup hummus (store-bought or homemade)

1 carrot, cut into sticks

1 cucumber, cut into sticks

1 red bell pepper, cut into sticks

1 yellow bell pepper, cut into sticks

1 stalk celery, cut into sticks

Nutritional Information (per serving):

Calories: 120

Protein: 3g

Carbohydrates: 12g

Dietary Fiber: 4g

Sugars: 3g

Fat: 7g

Saturated Fat: 1g

Sodium: 220mg

Preparation Steps:

1. Wash and Cut Vegetables: Rinse all the vegetables and cut them into sticks.

2. Arrange Veggie Sticks: Place the veggie sticks on a platter in a visually appealing way.

3. Serve Hummus: Put the hummus in a bowl and place it in the center of the platter.

4. Serve and Enjoy: Serve immediately, or cover and refrigerate until you're ready to snack!

Greek Yogurt Dip with Fresh Fruit

Description: A refreshing and light snack that pairs creamy Greek yogurt with fresh fruit. Rich in protein and probiotics, this snack supports digestion and overall well-being.

Prep Time: 10 minutes

Servings: 4

Ingredients:

1 cup Greek yogurt (plain, unsweetened)

1 tbsp honey

1/2 tsp vanilla extract

1 cup strawberries, hulled and halved

1 cup pineapple chunks

1 cup apple slices

1 cup grapes

Nutritional Information (per serving):

Calories: 130

Protein: 5g

Carbohydrates: 26g

Dietary Fiber: 3g

Sugars: 22g

Fat: 2g

Saturated Fat: 1g

Sodium: 30mg

Preparation Steps:

Mix Yogurt Dip: In a small bowl, combine Greek yogurt, honey, and vanilla extract. Mix until smooth.

Prepare Fruit: Wash and cut fresh fruit into bite-sized pieces.

Arrange Platter: Place fruit on a platter around the yogurt dip bowl.

Serve and Enjoy: Serve immediately, or cover and refrigerate until ready to eat.

Cheese and Crackers Platter

Description: A classic and elegant snack or appetizer that combines a variety of flavors and textures. Perfect for entertaining or a satisfying snack that's gentle on the digestive system.

Prep Time: 10 minutes

Servings: 4

Ingredients:

4 ounces cheddar cheese, sliced

4 ounces goat cheese, sliced

4 ounces mozzarella cheese, sliced

20 whole-grain crackers

1/4 cup dried apricots

1/4 cup almonds

Nutritional Information (per serving):

Calories: 250

Protein: 12g

Carbohydrates: 20g

Dietary Fiber: 3g

Sugars: 8g

Fat: 15g

Saturated Fat: 6g

Sodium: 300mg

Preparation Steps:

Arrange Cheese: Place slices of cheddar, goat, and mozzarella cheese on a platter.

Add Crackers: Arrange whole-grain crackers around the cheese.

Add Texture and Flavor: Add dried apricots and almonds to the platter.

Serve and Enjoy: Serve immediately, or cover and refrigerate until ready to eat.

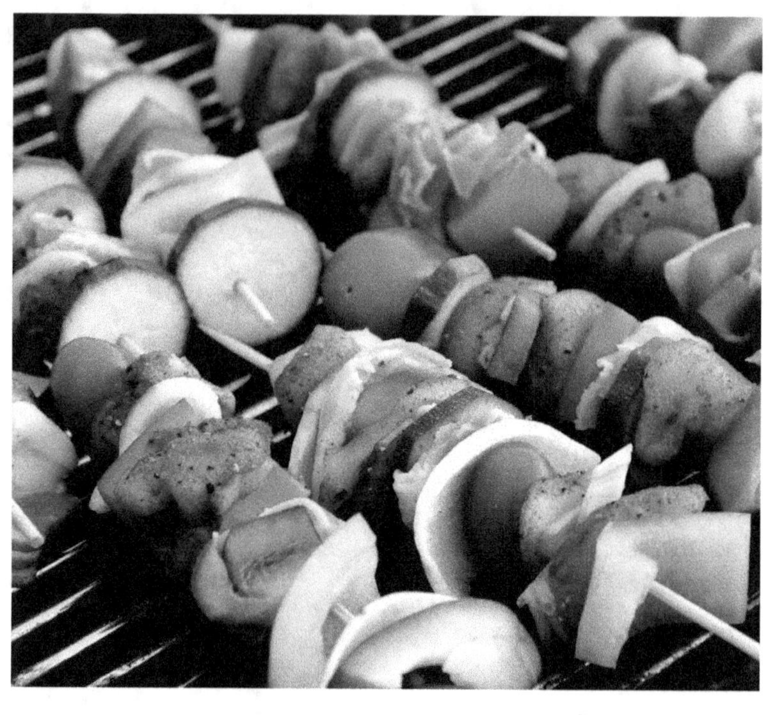

Caprese Skewers

Description: A delightful and elegant appetizer that combines fresh mozzarella, juicy cherry tomatoes, and fragrant basil. Perfect for any occasion, these bite-sized snacks are easy to prepare and packed with flavor.

Prep Time: 10 minutes

Servings: 4

Ingredients:

16 cherry tomatoes

16 small fresh mozzarella balls (bocconcini)

16 fresh basil leaves

2 tbsp balsamic glaze

1 tbsp olive oil

Salt and pepper to taste

16 small skewers or toothpicks

Nutritional Information (per serving):

Calories: 120

Protein: 6g

Carbohydrates: 3g

Dietary Fiber: 1g

Sugars: 2g

Fat: 10g

Saturated Fat: 3g

Sodium: 150mg

Preparation Steps:

1. Thread Skewers: Alternate cherry tomatoes, basil leaves, and mozzarella balls on each skewer.

2. Arrange Skewers: Place skewers on a serving platter.

3. Drizzle with Glaze: Drizzle with olive oil and balsamic glaze.

Season and serve with salt and pepper to taste. Serve immediately.

Trail Mix with Nuts and Dried Fruits

Description: A nutritious and energy-boosting homemade trail mix that combines a variety of nuts and dried fruits. Perfect for on-the-go snacking that's gentle on the gallbladder.

Prep Time: 5 minutes

Servings: 4

Ingredients:

1/2 cup almonds

1/2 cup cashews

1/2 cup walnuts

1/2 cup dried cranberries

1/2 cup dried apricots, chopped

1/4 cup pumpkin seeds

1/4 cup dark chocolate chips (optional)

Nutritional Information (per serving):

Calories: 250

Protein: 6g

Carbohydrates: 22g

Dietary Fiber: 4g

Sugars: 14g

Fat: 17g

Saturated Fat: 3g

Sodium: 5mg

Preparation Steps:

1. Combine the ingredients in a large bowl.

2. Mix Well: Ensure even distribution of ingredients.

3. Divide and Store: Divide into four portions and store in airtight containers.

4. Serve and Enjoy: Serve immediately or store for later use.

Stuffed Mini Peppers with Goat Cheese

Description: A delicious and colorful appetizer filled with creamy goat cheese and herbs. Perfect for entertaining, these stuffed mini peppers are a simple yet elegant snack.

Prep Time: 10 minutes

Servings: 4

Ingredients:

12 mini bell peppers

4 ounces goat cheese

1 tbsp fresh basil, finely chopped

1 tbsp fresh parsley, finely chopped

1 tsp lemon zest

Salt and pepper to taste

Olive oil for drizzling

Nutritional Information (per serving):

Calories: 130

Protein: 4g

Carbohydrates: 8g

Dietary Fiber: 2g

Sugars: 6g

Fat: 9g

Saturated Fat: 4g

Sodium: 150mg

Preparation Steps:

1. Prepare Peppers: Cut tops off mini bell peppers, and remove seeds.

2. Mix Goat Cheese Mixture: Combine goat cheese, basil, parsley, lemon zest, salt, and pepper.

3. Stuff Peppers: Fill each pepper with goat cheese mixture.

4. Arrange and Drizzle: Arrange stuffed peppers on a platter, and drizzle with olive oil.

Serve immediately or refrigerate until ready to use.

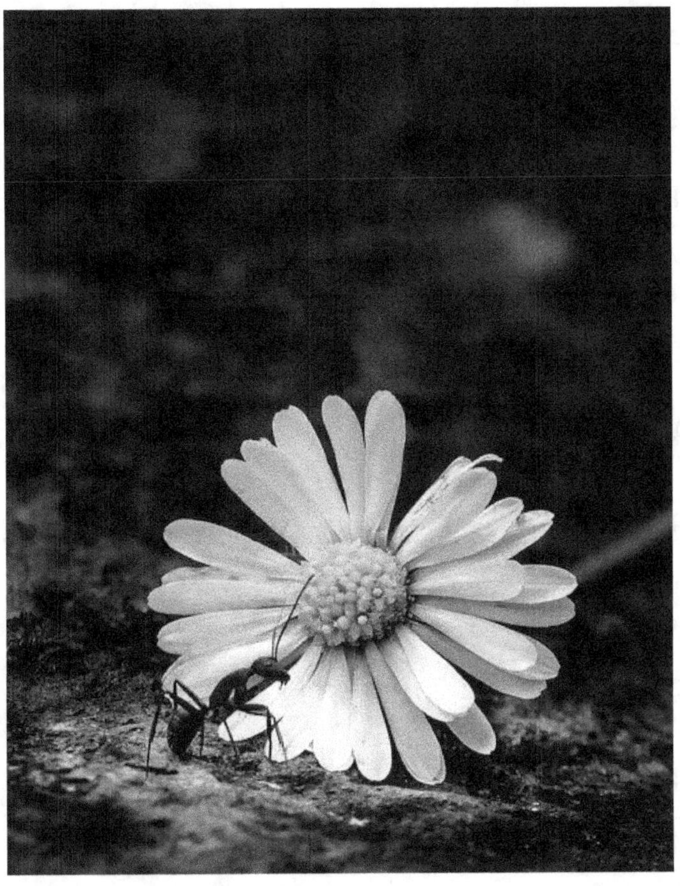

Ants on a Log

Description: A fun and nutritious snack that combines crisp celery with creamy peanut butter and sweet raisins. A delicious snack for kids and adults alike, offering a healthy balance of protein, healthy fats, and fiber.

Prep Time: 5 minutes

Servings: 4

Ingredients:

4 celery stalks

1/2 cup peanut butter (or other nut butter)

1/4 cup raisins

Nutritional Information (per serving):

Calories: 150

Protein: 4g

Carbohydrates: 18g

Dietary Fiber: 3g

Sugars: 11g

Fat: 9g

Saturated Fat: 2g

Sodium: 75mg

Preparation Steps:

1. Prepare Celery: Wash and cut celery stalks into 3-4 inch pieces.

2. Spread Peanut Butter: Generously spread peanut butter into the hollow of each celery piece.

3. Add Raisins: Place raisins on top of peanut butter, spaced evenly to resemble ants on a log.

4. Serve: Arrange on a plate and serve immediately

Guacamole and Salsa with Baked Tortilla Chips

Description: A classic and healthy snack or appetizer combo, providing healthy fats, fiber, and vitamins. Perfect for parties or a light snack.

Cooking Time: 10 minutes (for baking chips)

Prep Time: 10 minutes

Servings: 4

Ingredients:

Guacamole:

2 ripe avocados

1 small lime, juiced

1/4 cup red onion, finely chopped

1 small tomato, diced

1 tbsp fresh cilantro, chopped

1/2 tsp salt

1/4 tsp ground black pepper

Salsa:

2 ripe tomatoes, diced

1/4 cup red onion, finely chopped

1 jalapeño, seeded and finely chopped (optional)

1 tbsp fresh cilantro, chopped

1 small lime, juiced

1/2 tsp salt

1/4 tsp ground black pepper

Baked Tortilla Chips:

8 corn tortillas

1 tbsp olive oil

1/2 tsp salt

Nutritional Information (per serving):

Calories: 200

Protein: 4g

Carbohydrates: 24g

Dietary Fiber: 6g

Sugars: 2g

Fat: 12g

Saturated Fat: 2g

Sodium: 400mg

Preparation Steps:

Baked Tortilla Chips:

1. Preheat the oven to 350°F (175°C).

2. Cut tortillas into 6 triangles each.

3. Arrange on a baking sheet in a single layer.

4. Brush with olive oil and season with salt.

5. Bake for 10-12 minutes or until crisp and golden brown.

Let cool.

Guacamole:

1. Mash avocados in a medium bowl.

2. Add lime juice, red onion, tomato, cilantro, salt, and pepper.

3. Mix well and season to taste.

4. Transfer to a serving bowl.

Salsa:

Combine diced tomatoes, red onion, jalapeño (if using), cilantro, lime juice, salt, and pepper in a medium bowl.

Mix well and let sit for a few minutes to meld flavors.

Transfer to a serving bowl.

To Serve:

Arrange baked tortilla chips on a platter.

Serve with guacamole and salsa on the side.

CHAPTER 6:

SOUPS

Chicken Bone Broth

Description: A nourishing and comforting staple for anyone adapting to a no-gallbladder diet. Rich in minerals and collagen, essential for healing and digestion.

Cooking Time: 12 hours

Prep Time: 20 minutes

Servings: 8

Ingredients:

2 lbs chicken bones (preferably from organic, pasture-raised chickens)

2 medium carrots, roughly chopped

2 celery stalks, roughly chopped

1 large onion, quartered

4 cloves garlic, peeled

2 tablespoons apple cider vinegar

1 bay leaf

10-12 cups water

Salt and pepper to taste

Nutritional Information (per serving):

Calories: 80

Protein: 6g

Fat: 5g

Carbohydrates: 3g

Fiber: 1g

Preparation Steps:

Chicken Bone Broth:

Add Ingredients: Place chicken bones, carrots, celery, onion, and garlic in a large pot or slow cooker.

Add Water: Cover bones and vegetables with water by about 2 inches.

Add Bay Leaf: Put in the bay leaf.

Boil and Simmer: Bring to a gentle boil, then reduce heat to a low simmer.

Simmer: Cook for 12 hours, skimming off any foam or fat that rises to the top.

Strain: Strain broth through a fine mesh sieve, discarding solids. Season with salt and pepper to taste.

Cool and Refrigerate: Let broth cool, then refrigerate. Skim off solidified fat from the top before using.

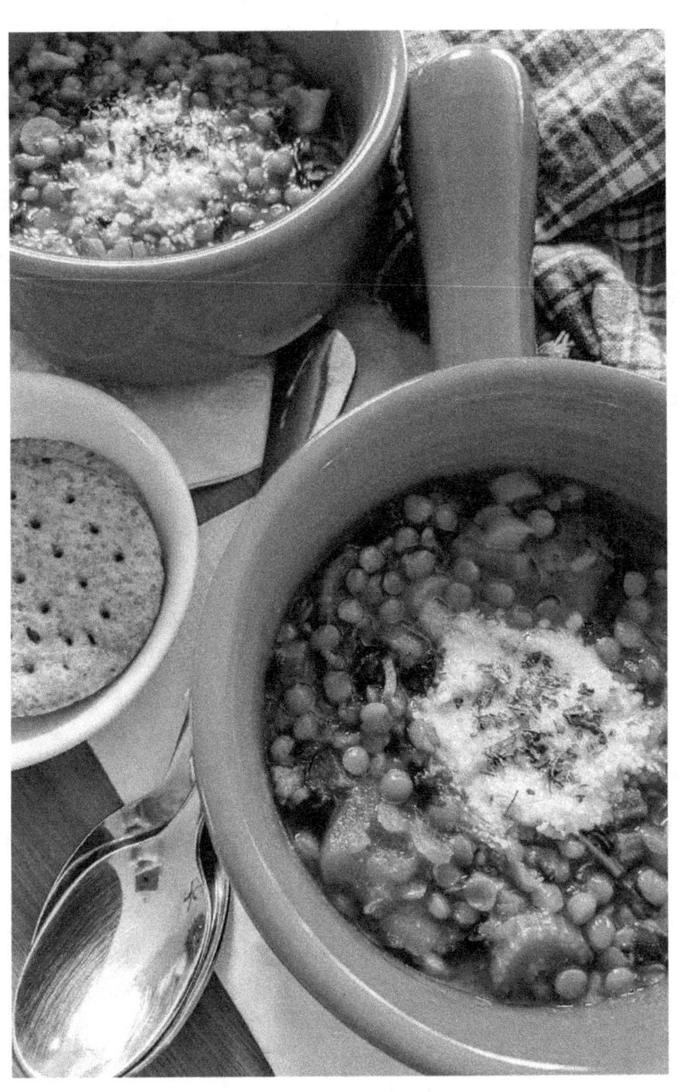

Vegetable Soup with Lentils

Description: A hearty and satisfying soup packed with fiber and plant-based protein from lentils, designed to gently soothe your digestive system while providing a robust and comforting meal.

Cooking Time: 45 minutes

Prep Time: 15 minutes

Servings: 6

Ingredients:

1 cup green or brown lentils, rinsed

2 tablespoons olive oil

1 large onion, diced

2 cloves garlic, minced

2 medium carrots, diced

2 celery stalks, diced

1 zucchini, diced

1 can (14.5 oz) diced tomatoes, with juice

6 cups low-sodium vegetable broth

1 teaspoon dried thyme

1 teaspoon ground cumin

2 cups chopped kale or spinach

Salt and pepper to taste

Juice of 1 lemon

Nutritional Information (per serving):

Calories: 210

Protein: 11g

Fat: 4g

Carbohydrates: 36g

Fiber: 15g

Preparation Steps:

Heat Oil: Heat olive oil in a large pot over medium heat.

Sauté Onion and Garlic: Cook until soft and translucent, about 5 minutes.

Add Vegetables: Add carrots, celery, and zucchini. Cook for another 5 minutes.

Add Lentils and Broth: Stir in lentils, diced tomatoes, vegetable broth, thyme, and cumin.

Simmer: Bring to a boil, then reduce heat and simmer for 30 minutes, or until lentils are tender.

Add Greens: Add kale or spinach and cook for another 5 minutes until wilted.

Season: Season with salt, pepper, and lemon juice.

Serve: Serve hot, with whole-grain bread if desired.

Miso Soup with Tofu and Seaweed

Description: A simple and flavorful miso soup, ideal for a light meal or starter, promoting healthy digestion with probiotics and essential nutrients from tofu and seaweed.

Cooking Time: 15 minutes

Prep Time: 10 minutes

Servings: 4

Ingredients:

4 cups water

1/4 cup miso paste (white or yellow)

1 cup silken tofu, cubed

1/4 cup dried wakame seaweed

2 green onions, thinly sliced

1 tablespoon soy sauce (optional)

1 teaspoon sesame oil (optional)

Nutritional Information (per serving):

Calories: 80

Protein: 6g

Fat: 3g

Carbohydrates: 8g

Fiber: 1g

Preparation Steps:

Simmer Water: Bring water to a gentle simmer in a medium pot.

Dissolve Miso: Dissolve miso paste with hot water, then stir back into the pot.

Add Tofu and Seaweed: Add tofu and wakame seaweed to the pot.

Simmer: Simmer for 5 minutes, until seaweed rehydrates and tofu is heated through.

Add Green Onions: Stir in green onions.

Add Optional Flavorings: Add soy sauce and sesame oil, if using, for additional flavor.

Serve: Serve immediately.

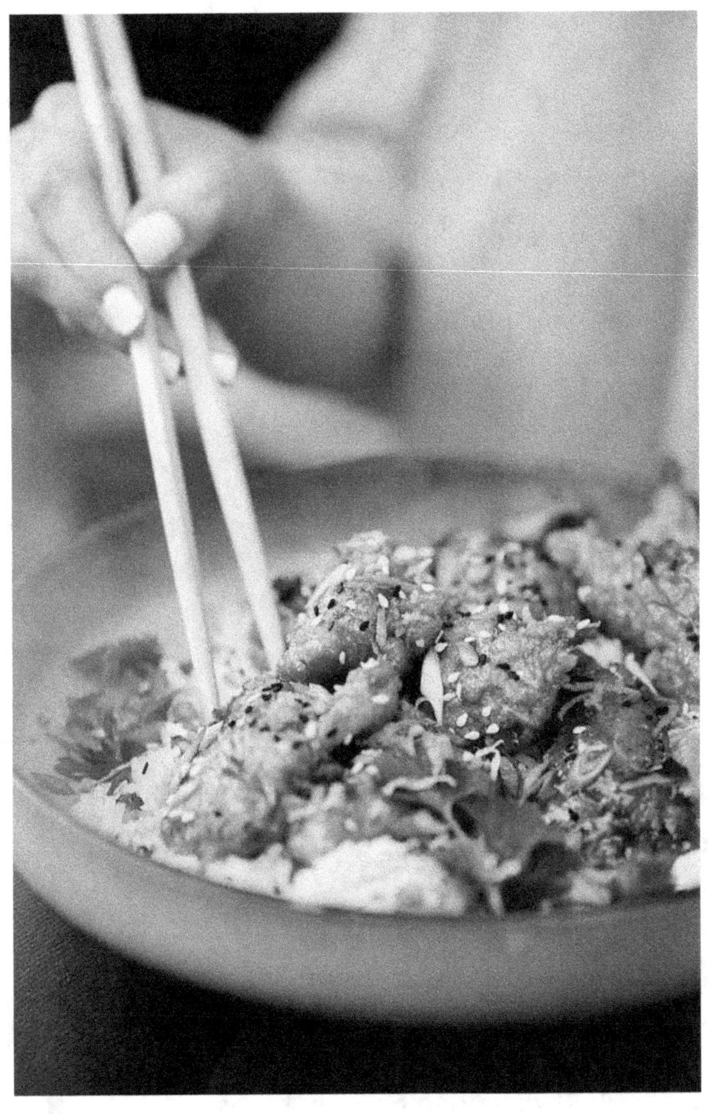

Chicken and Rice Soup

Description: A soothing, hearty meal that's light yet filling, with tender chicken, soft rice, and a medley of vegetables.

Cooking Time: 1 hour

Prep Time: 20 minutes

Servings: 6

Ingredients:

1 tablespoon olive oil

1 medium onion, diced

2 cloves garlic, minced

3 medium carrots, diced

2 celery stalks, diced

1 cup cooked shredded chicken breast

1 cup uncooked white rice

8 cups low-sodium chicken broth

1 bay leaf

1 teaspoon dried thyme

Salt and pepper to taste

2 tablespoons chopped fresh parsley (optional)

Nutritional Information (per serving):

Calories: 200

Protein: 15g

Fat: 5g

Carbohydrates: 25g

Fiber: 3g

Preparation Steps:

Heat Oil: Heat olive oil in a large pot over medium heat.

Sauté Onion and Garlic: Cook until soft and fragrant, about 5 minutes.

Add Carrots and Celery: Cook for another 5 minutes.

Add Chicken, Rice, and Broth: Add shredded chicken, rice, chicken broth, bay leaf, and thyme.

Bring to Boil and Simmer: Bring to a boil, then simmer for 25-30 minutes or until rice is tender.

Season and Serve: Remove bay leaf, season with salt and pepper, and stir in parsley (if using). Serve hot.

Beef and Barley Soup

Description: A robust and nutritious soup packed with tender beef, wholesome barley, and vegetables, providing an excellent source of protein and fiber for a satisfying meal.

Cooking Time: 1 hour 30 minutes

Prep Time: 20 minutes

Servings: 6

Ingredients:

1 lb beef stew meat, cut into small cubes

2 tablespoons olive oil

1 large onion, diced

2 cloves garlic, minced

3 medium carrots, diced

2 celery stalks, diced

1 cup pearl barley, rinsed

8 cups low-sodium beef broth

1 bay leaf

1 teaspoon dried thyme

Salt and pepper to taste

2 tablespoons chopped fresh parsley (optional)

Nutritional Information (per serving):

Calories: 350

Protein: 25g

Fat: 12g

Carbohydrates: 35g

Fiber: 8g

Preparation Steps:

Brown Beef: Heat olive oil in a large pot over medium heat. Add beef cubes and brown on all sides, about 5-7 minutes. Set aside.

Sauté Onion and Garlic: Cook until soft and fragrant, about 5 minutes.

Add Carrots and Celery: Cook for another 5 minutes.

Add Beef, Barley, and Broth: Stir in browned beef, barley, beef broth, bay leaf, and thyme. Bring to a boil, then simmer.

Cook: Cook for 1 hour, or until beef is tender and barley is cooked.

Season and Serve: Remove bay leaf, season with salt and pepper, and stir in parsley (if using). Serve hot.

Butternut Squash Soup

Description: A comforting and nutritious soup that's gentle on the digestive system, with a velvety smooth texture and a hint of spice to enhance the natural sweetness of the squash.

Cooking Time: 45 minutes

Prep Time: 15 minutes

Servings: 6

Ingredients:

1 large butternut squash, peeled, seeded, and cubed

2 tablespoons olive oil

1 medium onion, diced

2 cloves garlic, minced

4 cups low-sodium vegetable broth

1 teaspoon ground cumin

1/2 teaspoon ground cinnamon

Salt and pepper to taste

1/2 cup coconut milk (optional)

2 tablespoons chopped fresh cilantro (optional)

Nutritional Information (per serving):

Calories: 150

Protein: 2g

Fat: 8g

Carbohydrates: 20g

Fiber: 4g

Preparation Steps:

Sauté Onion and Garlic: Cook in olive oil until soft and fragrant, about 5 minutes.

Add Squash: Stir to coat with oil and mix with onion and garlic.

Add Broth: Pour in vegetable broth and bring to a boil.

Simmer: Reduce heat and cook for 30 minutes or until squash is tender.

Puree: Use an immersion blender or transfer to a blender and blend until smooth.

Add Spices: Stir in cumin, cinnamon, salt, and pepper.

Add Coconut Milk (optional): Stir well to combine.

Serve: Serve hot, garnished with fresh cilantro if desired.

Creamy Tomato Basil Soup

Description: A comforting and nutritious classic soup that's perfect for a light lunch or dinner, made with fresh basil and ripe tomatoes that are easy to digest.

Cooking Time: 30 minutes

Prep Time: 15 minutes

Servings: 4

Ingredients:

1 tbsp olive oil

1 medium onion, chopped

2 cloves garlic, minced

6 ripe tomatoes, chopped

2 cups low-sodium vegetable broth

1/2 cup fresh basil leaves, chopped

1/2 cup light coconut milk

Salt and pepper to taste

Nutritional Information (per serving):

Calories: 150

Protein: 3g

Fat: 7g

Carbohydrates: 20g

Fiber: 4g

Preparation Steps:

Sauté Onion and Garlic: Heat olive oil and cook until soft and fragrant, about 5 minutes.

Add Tomatoes: Cook for another 5 minutes until they break down.

Add Broth: Pour in vegetable broth and bring to a simmer. Cook for 15 minutes.

Add Basil and Coconut Milk: Stir in fresh basil and coconut milk.

Using an immersion blender, purée the soup until smooth.

Season and serve with salt and pepper to taste.

Serve hot and garnish with fresh basil leaves.

Potato Leek Soup

Description: A hearty and comforting soup that's creamy without heavy cream, with leeks providing a subtle sweetness and potatoes giving it a rich texture, making it perfect for any season.

Cooking Time: 40 minutes

Prep Time: 15 minutes

Servings: 4

Ingredients:

2 tbsp olive oil

4 large leeks, white and light green parts only, sliced

3 cloves garlic, minced

4 medium potatoes, peeled and diced

4 cups low-sodium vegetable broth

1 cup unsweetened almond milk

Salt and pepper to taste

Chopped chives for garnish

Nutritional Information (per serving):

Calories: 180

Protein: 4g

Fat: 8g

Carbohydrates: 26g

Fiber: 4g

Preparation Steps:

Sauté Leeks and Garlic: Heat olive oil and cook until soft and translucent, about 10 minutes.

Cook Potatoes: Bring potatoes and vegetable broth to a boil, then simmer for 20 minutes or until tender.

Blend Soup: Use an immersion blender to blend until smooth.

Add Almond Milk and Season: Stir in almond milk and season with salt and pepper.

Heat and Serve: Heat gently until warmed through. Serve hot, garnished with chopped chives.

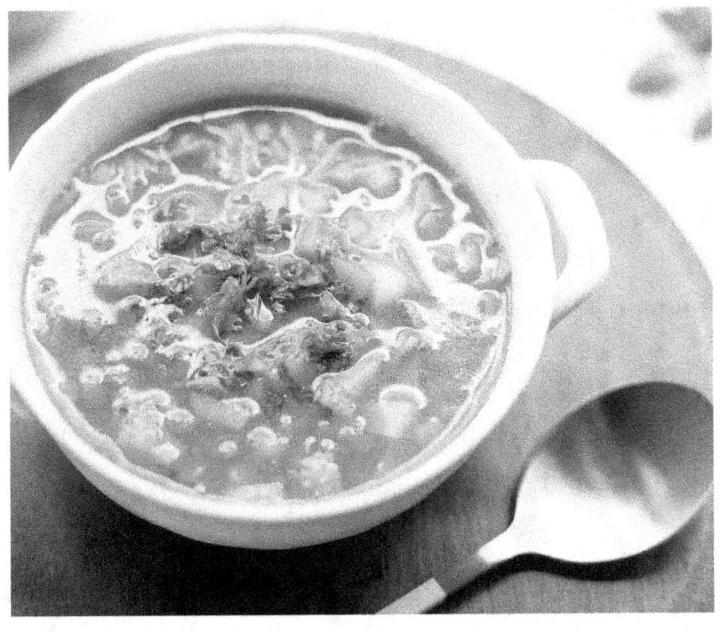

Minestrone Soup

Description: A versatile and nutrient-rich soup that can be enjoyed year-round, adapted to seasonal ingredients, and packed with flavor.

Cooking Time: 45 minutes

Prep Time: 20 minutes

Servings: 6

Ingredients:

2 tbsp olive oil

1 medium onion, chopped

2 cloves garlic, minced

2 carrots, diced

2 celery stalks, diced

1 zucchini, diced

1 can (15 oz) diced tomatoes

4 cups low-sodium vegetable broth

1 can (15 oz) of cannellini beans, drained and rinsed

1 cup small pasta (like ditalini or elbow)

2 cups spinach leaves

1 tsp dried oregano

Salt and pepper to taste

Nutritional Information (per serving):

Calories: 220

Protein: 8g

Fat: 6g

Carbohydrates: 35g

Fiber: 8g

Preparation Steps:

Sauté Onion and Garlic: Cook in olive oil until soft and fragrant, about 5 minutes.

Add Vegetables: Cook carrots, celery, and zucchini until softened, about 5 minutes.

Add Tomatoes and Broth: Stir in diced tomatoes and vegetable broth. Bring to a boil, then let it simmer for 20 minutes.

Cook Pasta and Beans: Add cannellini beans and pasta. Cook for approximately 10 minutes, or until the pasta is al dente.

Season and Serve: Combine spinach, oregano, salt, and pepper

 Serve

Thai Coconut Curry Soup

Description: A delightful fusion of flavors, featuring a fragrant coconut curry broth, tender vegetables, and fresh lime, making for a light and satisfying meal that's gentle on the digestive system.

Cooking Time: 30 minutes

Prep Time: 15 minutes

Servings: 4

Ingredients:

1 tbsp olive oil

1 medium onion, chopped

1 red bell pepper, sliced

1 cup mushrooms, sliced

2 cloves garlic, minced

1 tbsp grated ginger

1 tbsp red curry paste

1 can (14 oz) light coconut milk

3 cups low-sodium vegetable broth

1 cup baby spinach

1 tbsp lime juice

Fresh cilantro for garnish

Nutritional Information (per serving):

Calories: 190

Protein: 4g

Fat: 12g

Carbohydrates: 18g

Fiber: 4g

Preparation Steps:

Sauté Vegetables: Heat olive oil and cook until soft, about 5 minutes.

Add Aromatics: Add garlic and ginger and cook for another minute.

Add Curry Paste: Stir in red curry paste and cook for 1 minute.

Simmer Broth: Pour in coconut milk and vegetable broth. Simmer for 10 minutes.

Add Spinach and Lime Juice: Stir in baby spinach and lime juice. Serve hot, garnished with fresh cilantro.

CHAPTER 7:

VEGAN AND VEGETARIAN MAINS

In this chapter, we delve into the world of plant-based cuisine, exploring a variety of delicious and innovative vegan and vegetarian main course options. From hearty bowls to flavorful stir-fries, these recipes showcase the rich flavors and textures of plant-based ingredients, perfect for vegetarians and vegans alike. Get ready to inspire your taste buds and nourish your body with these wholesome and satisfying dishes.

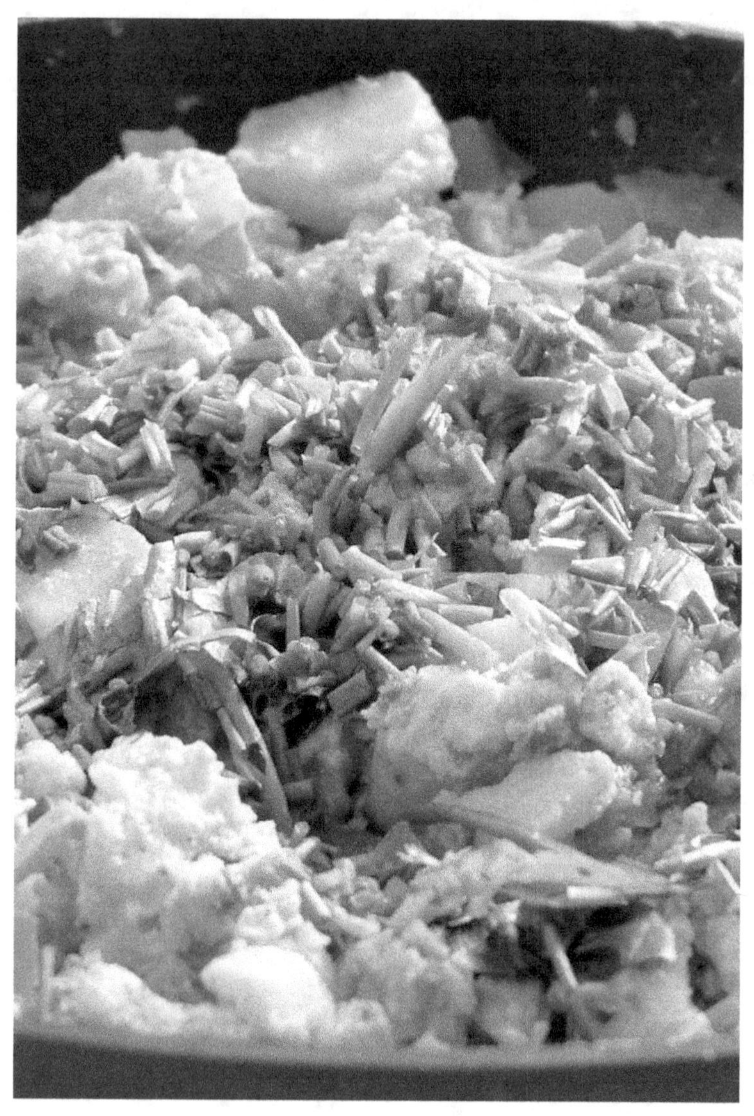

Lentil and Vegetable Stir-Fry

Description: A quick and satisfying vegan main dish packed with protein-rich lentils and a variety of fresh vegetables, perfect for lunch or dinner.

Cooking Time: 25 minutes

Prep Time: 15 minutes

Servings: 4

Ingredients:

1 cup dried green or brown lentils, washed and drained

2 tbsp olive oil

1 medium onion, sliced

2 cloves of garlic, minced

1 red bell pepper, sliced

1 yellow bell pepper, sliced

1 zucchini, sliced

1 cup broccoli florets

2 tbsp soy sauce (low sodium)

1 tbsp rice vinegar

1 tsp sesame oil

1 tbsp sesame seeds

Fresh cilantro for garnish

Nutritional Information (per serving):

Calories: 320

Protein: 14g

Fat: 10g

Carbohydrates: 46g

Fiber: 16g

Preparation Steps:

Cook Lentils: Boil lentils until tender, about 15-20 minutes. Drain and set aside.

Sauté Aromatics: Heat olive oil and sauté onion and garlic until fragrant, about 2 minutes.

Stir-Fry Vegetables: Add bell peppers, zucchini, and broccoli. Stir-fry for 5-7 minutes, until tender-crisp.

Combine Lentils and Vegetables: Stir in cooked lentils, soy sauce, rice vinegar, and sesame oil. Cook for another 2-3 minutes.

Serve: Sprinkle with sesame seeds and garnish with fresh cilantro. Serve hot.

Chickpea Curry with Spinach

Description: A creamy and nutritious curry made with chickpeas, spinach, and a blend of warm spices, served over rice or quinoa for a wholesome meal.

Cooking Time: 30 minutes

Prep Time: 15 minutes

Servings: 4

Ingredients:

2 tbsp olive oil

1 medium onion, chopped

3 cloves garlic, minced

1 tbsp grated ginger

1 tbsp curry powder

1 tsp ground cumin

1 tsp ground turmeric

1 can (15 oz) of chickpeas, drained and rinsed

1 can (14 oz) light coconut milk

1 cup low-sodium vegetable broth

4 cups fresh spinach

1 tbsp lime juice

Salt and pepper to taste

Fresh cilantro for garnish

Nutritional Information (per serving):

Calories: 280

Protein: 9g

Fat: 16g

Carbohydrates: 28g

Fiber: 8g

Preparation Steps:

Sauté Aromatics: Heat olive oil and cook onion, garlic, and ginger until soft, about 5 minutes.

Toast Spices: Stir in curry powder, cumin, and turmeric. Cook for 1 minute.

Simmer Curry: Add chickpeas, coconut milk, and vegetable broth. Cook for 15 minutes.

Add Spinach: Stir in fresh spinach and lime juice. Cook until the spinach has wilted, which should take about 2-3 minutes.

Season and Serve: Season with salt and pepper. Serve hot, garnished with fresh cilantro.

Vegan Chili

Description: A hearty and robust vegan chili packed with beans, vegetables, and spices, perfect for a cozy dinner.

Cooking Time: 45 minutes

Prep Time: 20 minutes

Servings: 6

Ingredients:

2 tbsp olive oil

1 large onion, chopped

3 cloves of garlic, minced

2 carrots, diced

2 celery stalks, diced

1 red bell pepper, chopped

1 green bell pepper, chopped

1 can (15 oz) of black beans, drained and rinsed

1 can (15 oz) kidney beans, drained and rinsed

1 can (15 oz) diced tomatoes

2 cups low-sodium vegetable broth

2 tbsp tomato paste

1 tbsp chili powder

1 tsp ground cumin

1 tsp smoked paprika

1/2 tsp cayenne pepper (optional, for heat)

Salt and pepper to taste

Fresh cilantro and avocado slices for garnish

Nutritional Information (per serving):

Calories: 310

Protein: 12g

Fat: 8g

Carbohydrates: 48g

Fiber: 14g

Preparation Steps:

Sauté Aromatics: Heat olive oil and cook onion and garlic until soft, about 5 minutes.

Add Vegetables: Cook carrots, celery, and bell peppers until tender, about 5-7 minutes.

Add Beans and Spices: Stir in black beans, kidney beans, diced tomatoes, vegetable broth, tomato paste, chili powder, cumin, smoked paprika, and cayenne pepper (if using).

Simmer Chili: Bring to a simmer and cook for 20-25 minutes, allowing flavors to blend.

Season and Serve: Season with salt and pepper. Serve hot, garnished with fresh cilantro and avocado slices.

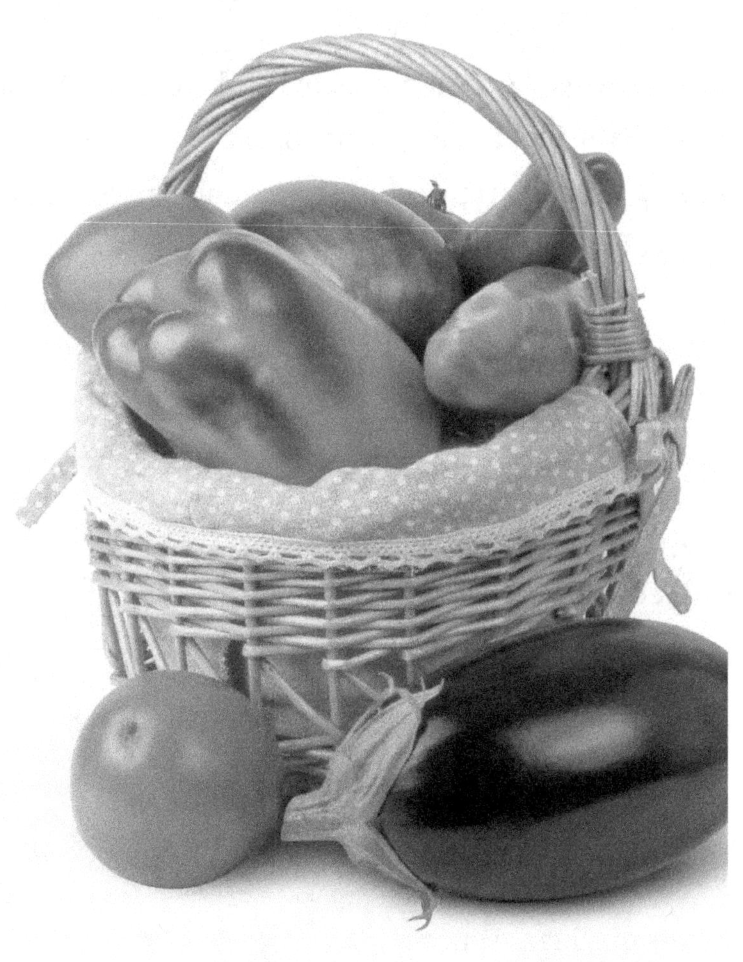

Eggplant Parmesan

Description: A vegan version of the classic Italian dish, featuring breaded and baked eggplant slices layered with marinara sauce and dairy-free cheese, perfect for a satisfying dinner.

Cooking Time: 60 minutes

Prep Time: 20 minutes

Servings: 4

Ingredients:

2 large eggplants, sliced into 1/2-inch rounds

1 cup almond flour

1 cup unsweetened almond milk

2 cups marinara sauce

1 cup dairy-free mozzarella cheese, shredded

1/2 cup nutritional yeast

1 tsp dried oregano

1 tsp garlic powder

Salt and pepper to taste

Fresh basil leaves for garnish

Nutritional Information (per serving):

Calories: 350

Protein: 12g

Fat: 18g

Carbohydrates: 38g

Fiber: 12g

Preparation Steps:

Prepare Eggplant: Dip eggplant slices in almond milk, then coat with almond flour mixture. Place on a baking sheet.

Bake Eggplant: Bake for 20 minutes, flipping halfway, until golden and tender.

Assemble Parmesan: Layer eggplant slices with marinara sauce, dairy-free mozzarella, and nutritional yeast in a baking dish.

Bake Parmesan: Bake for another 20-25 minutes until bubbly and golden.

Garnish and serve with fresh basil leaves.

Tofu Scramble with Veggies

Description: A versatile and protein-packed dish, this tofu scramble is a tasty alternative to scrambled eggs. Mixed with colorful vegetables and aromatic spices, it's an excellent choice for breakfast or brunch.

Cooking Time: 15 minutes Prep Time: 10 minutes Servings: 2 Ingredients:

1 block (14 oz) firm tofu, drained and crumbled 1 tbsp olive oil

1 small onion, chopped

1 red bell pepper, diced

1 zucchini, diced

2 cloves garlic, minced

1 tsp turmeric powder

1 tsp ground cumin

1 tbsp nutritional yeast of Scramble with Veggies

Salt and pepper to taste

Fresh parsley for garnish

Nutritional Information (per serving):

Calories: 250 Protein: 20g

Fat: 14g Carbohydrates: 18g Fiber: 5g

Preparation Steps:

In a large skillet, heat olive oil over medium heat. Add the onion and garlic, and sauté until translucent, about 3 minutes.

Cook the bell pepper and zucchini until soft, about 5 minutes.

Stir in the crumbled tofu, turmeric, cumin, nutritional yeast, salt, and pepper. Cook for a another 5-7 minutes, until thoroughly cooked and well mixed.

Garnish with fresh parsley and serve hot.

Tofu Scramble with Veggies

Description: A protein-packed and versatile dish, this tofu scramble is a delicious alternative to scrambled eggs, perfect for breakfast or brunch.

Cooking Time: 15 minutes

Prep Time: 10 minutes

Servings: 2

Ingredients:

1 block (14 oz) firm tofu, drained and crumbled

1 tbsp olive oil

1 small onion, chopped

1 red bell pepper, diced

1 zucchini, diced

2 cloves garlic, minced

1 tsp turmeric powder

1 tsp ground cumin

1 tbsp nutritional yeast

Salt and pepper to taste

Fresh parsley for garnish

Nutritional Information (per serving):

Calories: 250

Protein: 20g

Fat: 14g

Carbohydrates: 18g

Fiber: 5g

Preparation Steps:

Sauté Aromatics: Heat olive oil and cook onion and garlic until translucent, about 3 minutes.

Add Vegetables: Cook bell pepper and zucchini until tender, about 5 minutes.

Add Tofu and Spices: Stir in tofu, turmeric, cumin, nutritional yeast, salt, and pepper. Cook for 5-7 minutes until heated through.

Garnish and Serve: Sprinkle with fresh parsley and serve hot.

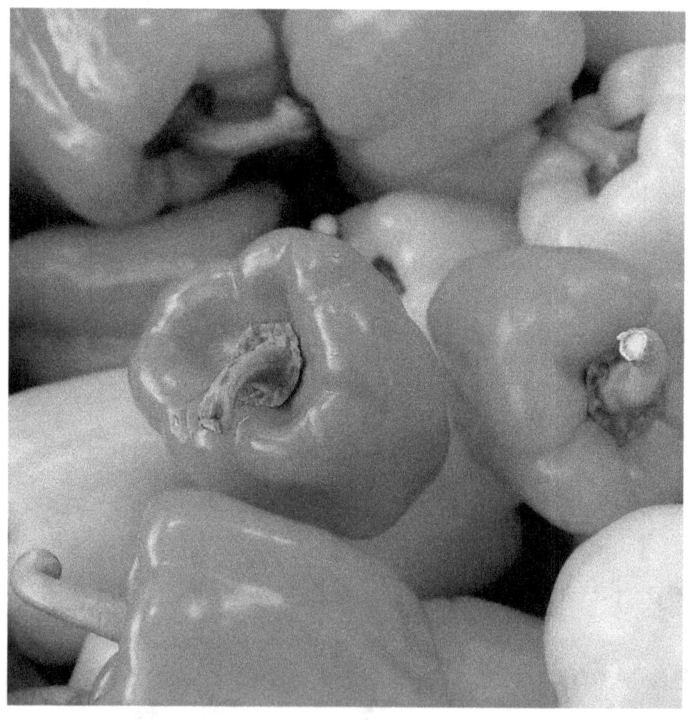

Quinoa Stuffed Bell Peppers

Description: A nutrient-dense and flavorful meal, these quinoa-stuffed bell peppers are filled with a delicious mix of quinoa, vegetables, and herbs, making a beautiful presentation perfect for a healthy dinner.

Cooking Time: 40 minutes

Prep Time: 20 minutes

Servings: 4

Ingredients:

4 large bell peppers, trimmed and seeds removed

1 cup quinoa, rinsed and drained

2 cups low-sodium vegetable broth

1 tbsp olive oil

1 small onion, chopped

2 cloves of garlic, minced

1 cup cherry tomatoes, halved

1 cup spinach, chopped

1 tsp dried oregano

1 tsp smoked paprika

Salt and pepper to taste

Fresh parsley for garnish

Nutritional Information (per serving):

Calories: 300

Protein: 10g

Fat: 10g

Carbohydrates: 44g

Fiber: 9g

Preparation Steps:

Prepare Bell Peppers: Place bell peppers in a baking dish.

Cook Quinoa: Simmer the quinoa in vegetable broth until cooked and absorbed.

Sauté Vegetables: Cook onion, garlic, cherry tomatoes, spinach, oregano, smoked paprika, salt, and pepper in olive oil.

Mix Quinoa and Vegetables: Combine cooked quinoa with vegetable mixture.

Stuff Bell Peppers: Spoon mixture into bell peppers.

Cover with foil and bake for 30 minutes. Remove the foil and bake for an additional 10 minutes.

Garnish and Serve: Sprinkle with fresh parsley and serve hot.

Black Bean and Sweet Potato Enchiladas

Description: A comforting and nutritious meal, these black bean and sweet potato enchiladas are topped with enchilada sauce and dairy-free cheese, perfect for an evening meal.

Cooking Time: 45 minutes

Prep Time: 20 minutes

Servings: 4

Ingredients:

2 medium sweet potatoes, peeled and diced

1 can (15 oz) of black beans, drained and rinsed

1 small onion, chopped

2 cloves garlic, minced

1 tbsp olive oil

1 tsp ground cumin

1 tsp chili powder

8 small corn tortillas

2 cups enchilada sauce

1 cup dairy-free cheese, shredded

Fresh cilantro for garnish

Nutritional Information (per serving):

Calories: 350

Protein: 10g

Fat: 10g

Carbohydrates: 60g

Fiber: 12g

Preparation Steps:

Sauté Onion and Garlic: Heat olive oil and cook until soft, about 5 minutes.

Add Sweet Potatoes and Spices: Cook until sweet potatoes are tender, about 10 minutes.

Stir in Black Beans: Cook for another 5 minutes until heated through.

Warm Tortillas: Make them pliable.

Assemble Enchiladas: Fill tortillas with sweet potato and black bean mixture, roll up, and place in baking dish.

Top with Enchilada Sauce and Cheese: Pour sauce and sprinkle cheese.Cover with foil and bake for 20 minutes.

Remove foil and bake for another 10 minutes until cheese is melted and bubbly.

Garnish and Serve: Garnish with fresh cilantro and serve hot.

Ratatouille

Description: Ratatouille is a classic French vegetable stew that showcases colorful and flavorful vegetables. This dish is both light and satisfying, making it great for a healthy and vibrant meal.

Cooking Time: 1 hour

Prep Time: 20 minutes

Servings: 4

Ingredients:

2 tbsp olive oil

1 large onion, chopped

3 cloves garlic, minced

1 eggplant, diced

2 zucchinis, sliced

1 red bell pepper, chopped

1 yellow bell pepper, chopped

4 tomatoes, chopped

1 tsp dried thyme

1 tsp dried basil

Salt and pepper to taste

Fresh basil leaves for garnish

Nutritional Information (per serving):

Calories: 200

Protein: 4g

Fat: 10g

Carbohydrates: 28g

Fiber: 10g

Preparation Steps:

Sauté Onion and Garlic: Heat olive oil and cook until soft, about 5 minutes.

Add Eggplant: Cook for 5-7 minutes until it softens.

Add Remaining Vegetables and Herbs: Stir in zucchini, bell peppers, tomatoes, thyme, and basil. Season with salt and pepper.

Simmer and Cook: Bring to a simmer, then reduce heat to low and cover. Cook for 30-40 minutes, stirring occasionally, until all vegetables are tender and flavors are well blended.

Adjust Seasoning and Serve: Adjust seasoning as needed. Serve hot and garnish with fresh basil leaves.

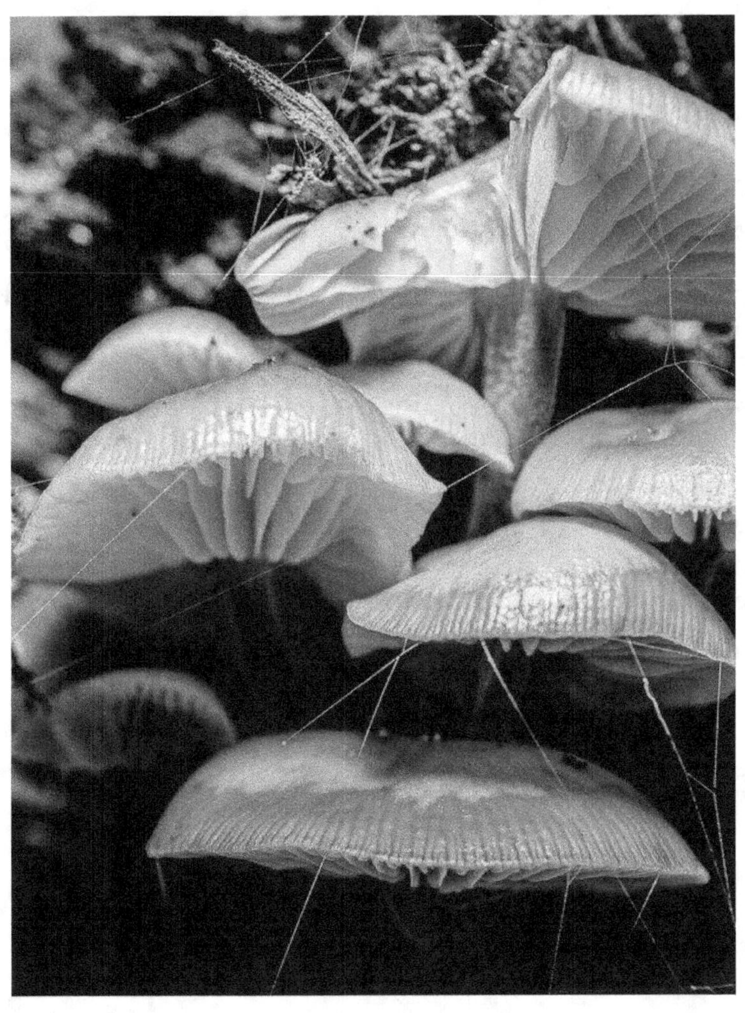

Mushroom Risotto

Description: A rich and indulgent dish, this creamy mushroom risotto requires no dairy. The combination of earthy mushrooms and perfectly cooked Arborio rice makes for a comforting and elegant meal.

Cooking Time: 40 minutes

Prep Time: 15 minutes

Servings: 4

Ingredients:

2 tbsp olive oil

1 small onion, finely chopped

2 cloves garlic, minced

2 cups Arborio rice

4 cups low-sodium vegetable broth, warmed

1 cup dry white wine (optional)

2 cups mushrooms, sliced

1 tbsp nutritional yeast

Salt and pepper to taste

Fresh parsley for garnish

Nutritional Information (per serving):

Calories: 350

Protein: 7g

Fat: 10g

Carbohydrates: 55g

Fiber: 3g

Preparation Steps:

Sauté Onion and Garlic: Heat olive oil and cook until translucent, about 5 minutes.

Add Mushrooms: Cook until they release their moisture and brown, about 5-7 minutes.

Add Arborio Rice: Cook for 2 minutes until lightly toasted.

Add White Wine (optional): Stir until absorbed.

Add Vegetable Broth: Gradually add, stirring frequently, allowing liquid to be absorbed before adding more.

Cook Until Creamy: Continue the process until rice is creamy and cooked through about 20-25 minutes.

Stir in Nutritional Yeast: Season with salt and pepper. Serve hot, garnished with fresh parsley.

Spaghetti Squash with Marinara Sauce

Description: A delicious low-carb alternative to pasta, spaghetti squash is paired with a robust marinara sauce for a light and flavorful healthy meal.

Cooking Time: 45 minutes

Prep Time: 10 minutes

Servings: 4

Ingredients:

1 large spaghetti squash

2 tbsp olive oil

1 small onion, chopped

3 cloves garlic, minced

1 can (28 oz) crushed tomatoes

1 tsp dried oregano

1 tsp dried basil

Salt and pepper to taste

Fresh basil leaves for garnish

Nutritional Information (per serving):

Calories: 180

Protein: 3g

Fat: 10g

Carbohydrates: 24g

Fiber: 5g

Preparation Steps:

Roast Spaghetti Squash: Preheat oven to 400°F(200°C). Cut squash in half lengthwise, remove seeds, and roast for 30-40 minutes until tender.

Sauté Onion and Garlic: Heat olive oil in a large skillet over medium heat. Cook the onion and garlic for about 5 minutes, or until they are tender.

Simmer Marinara Sauce: Stir in crushed tomatoes, oregano, basil, salt, and pepper. Simmer for 15-20 minutes until the sauce thickens and flavors meld.

Scrape Out Squash Flesh: Use a fork to scrape out flesh into spaghetti-like strands.

Serve Top squash with marinara sauce and garnish with fresh basil leaves.

CHAPTER 8:

SAVORY MEAT-BASED DISHES

In this chapter, we indulge in the rich flavors and textures of savory meat-based dishes, showcasing a range of mouthwatering recipes that are sure to satisfy any meat lover's cravings. From tender steaks to flavorful stews, and from juicy burgers to succulent roasts, these recipes highlight the versatility and richness of meat in all its forms. Get ready to fire up your grill, sharpen your knives, and delight in the hearty flavors of these savory meat-based dishes.

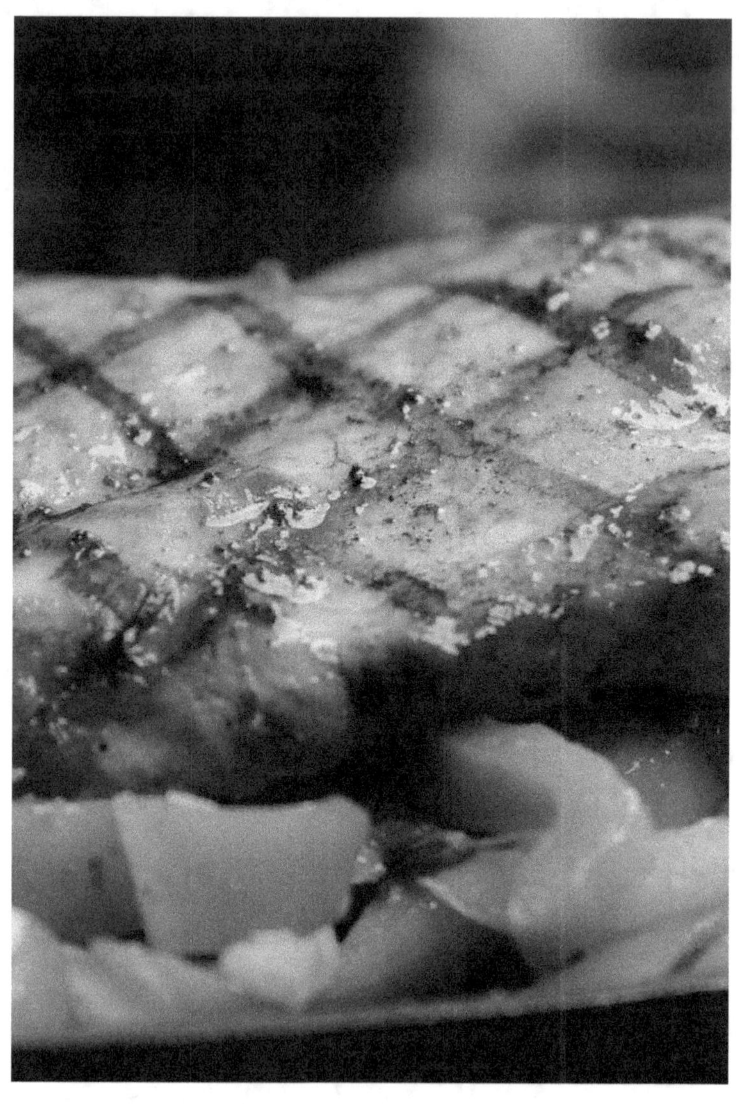

Grilled Chicken Breast with Lemon and Herbs

Description: Tender and flavorful grilled chicken breast, marinated with lemon and herbs, perfect for any meal. Serve with steamed vegetables or a light salad for a balanced meal.

Cooking Time: 20 minutes

Prep Time: 10 minutes (plus 30 minutes for marinating)

Servings: 4

Ingredients:

4 boneless, skinless chicken breasts

1/4 cup olive oil

1/4 cup fresh lemon juice

2 cloves garlic, minced

1 tbsp fresh rosemary, chopped

1 tbsp fresh thyme, chopped

Salt and pepper to taste

Lemon wedges for serving

Nutritional Information (per serving):

Calories: 250

Protein: 30g

Fat: 14g

Carbohydrates: 2g

Fiber: 0g

Preparation Steps:

Prepare Marinade: Whisk together olive oil, lemon juice, garlic, rosemary, thyme, salt, and pepper.

Marinate Chicken: Place chicken breasts in a resealable plastic bag or shallow dish. Pour marinade over chicken, coating well. Marinate in the refrigerator for a minimum of 30 minutes.

Grill Chicken: Preheat the grill to medium-high heat. Take the chicken out of the marinade. Grill chicken for 6-7 minutes on each side, or until internal temperature reaches 165°F (74°C).

Serve: Serve hot, garnished with lemon wedges.

Baked Salmon with Dill Sauce

Description: A simple and nutritious dish featuring baked salmon elevated by a creamy dill sauce, perfect for a quick and healthy weeknight dinner.

Cooking Time: 20 minutes

Prep Time: 10 minutes

Servings: 4

Ingredients:

4 salmon filets (about 6 oz each)

2 tbsp olive oil

Salt and pepper to taste

1/2 cup plain Greek yogurt

2 tbsp fresh dill, chopped

1 tbsp lemon juice

1 tsp lemon zest

1 clove garlic, minced

Nutritional Information (per serving):

Calories: 320

Protein: 34g

Fat: 18g

Carbohydrates: 2g

Fiber: 0g

Preparation Steps:

Preheat Oven: Preheat oven to 400°F (200°C). Prepare a baking sheet with parchment paper.

Prepare Salmon: Place salmon filets on the prepared baking sheet. Drizzle with olive oil, then season with salt and pepper.

Bake Salmon: Bake for 15-20 minutes, or until salmon flakes easily with a fork.

Prepare Dill Sauce: Mix Greek yogurt, dill, lemon juice, lemon zest, and garlic in a small bowl.

Serve: Serve salmon hot, topped with the dill sauce.

Turkey Meatballs in Marinara Sauce

Description: A healthier alternative to traditional meatballs, these baked turkey meatballs are simmered in marinara sauce for a delicious and comforting meal.

Cooking Time: 40 minutes

Prep Time: 15 minutes

Servings: 4

Ingredients:

1 lb ground turkey

1/4 cup almond flour

1 egg, beaten

1/4 cup fresh parsley, chopped

2 cloves garlic, minced

1 tsp dried oregano

1/2 tsp salt

1/4 tsp black pepper

2 cups marinara sauce

Fresh basil for garnish

Nutritional Information (per serving):

Calories: 280

Protein: 25g

Fat: 15g

Carbohydrates: 10g

Fiber: 3g

Preparation Steps:

Preheat Oven: Preheat oven to 375°F (190°C). Prepare a baking sheet with parchment paper.

Mix Meatball Mixture: Combine ground turkey, almond flour, egg, parsley, garlic, oregano, salt, and pepper in a large bowl.

Form Meatballs: Form mixture into 1-inch meatballs and place on prepared baking sheet.

Bake Meatballs: Bake for 20-25 minutes, or until cooked through and golden brown.

Simmer in Marinara Sauce: Heat marinara sauce in a large saucepan over medium heat. Add meatballs and simmer for 10 minutes.

Serve: Serve hot, garnished with fresh basil.

Beef Stir-Fry with Broccoli and Bell Peppers

Description: A quick and easy beef stir-fry packed with colorful vegetables, featuring tender strips of beef, crunchy broccoli, and peppers, making a flavorful and nutritious meal.

Cooking Time: 20 minutes

Prep Time: 15 minutes

Servings: 4

Ingredients:

1 lb beef sirloin, thinly sliced

2 tbsp soy sauce (or tamari for gluten-free)

1 tbsp cornstarch

2 tbsp vegetable oil, divided

1 small onion, thinly sliced

2 cloves garlic, minced

1 large broccoli head, cut into florets

1 red bell pepper, thinly sliced

1 yellow bell pepper, thinly sliced

1/4 cup low-sodium beef broth

1 tbsp oyster sauce (optional)

1 tsp sesame oil

1 tsp grated fresh ginger

Sesame seeds and chopped green onions for garnish

Nutritional Information (per serving):

Calories: 320

Protein: 28g

Fat: 18g

Carbohydrates: 12g

Fiber: 3g

Preparation Steps:

Marinate Beef: Toss sliced beef with soy sauce and cornstarch. Set aside.

Cook Beef: Heat 1 tbsp of vegetable oil in a large skillet or wok over medium-high heat. Add beef and stir-fry until browned and cooked through, about 4-5 minutes. Remove and set aside.

Sauté Onion and Garlic: Heat remaining oil. Sauté the onion and garlic until aromatic, about 2 minutes.

Stir-Fry Vegetables: Add broccoli and bell peppers. Stir-fry until tender-crisp, about 5-7 minutes.

Return Beef and Add Sauce: Return beef to skillet. Add beef broth, oyster sauce (if using), sesame oil, and grated ginger. Stir well and cook for another 2 minutes until heated through.

Garnish and Serve: Garnish with sesame seeds and chopped green onions before serving.

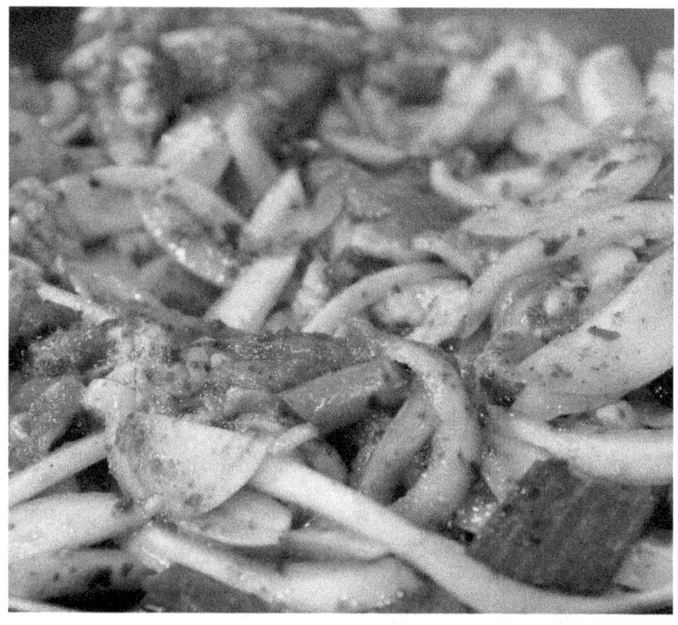

Turkey and Veggie Stir-Fry

Description: A simple and healthy stir-fry featuring ground turkey, savory sauce, and colorful vegetables, full of fresh flavors and bright colors.

Cooking Time: 20 minutes

Prep Time: 15 minutes

Servings: 4

Ingredients:

1 lb ground turkey

2 tablespoons soy sauce (or tamari if gluten-free)

1 tbsp olive oil

1 small onion, chopped

2 cloves garlic, minced

1 cup snap peas, trimmed

1 red bell pepper, sliced

1 yellow bell pepper, sliced

1 carrot, julienned

1 tbsp rice vinegar

1 tbsp hoisin sauce

1 tsp sesame oil

1 tsp grated fresh ginger

Chopped fresh cilantro for garnish

Nutritional Information (per serving):

Calories: 280

Protein: 25g

Fat: 14g

Carbohydrates: 15g

Fiber: 3g

Preparation Steps:

Cook Turkey: Heat olive oil in a large skillet or wok over medium-high heat. Add ground turkey and heat until browned, Break it up with a spoon for around 5-7 minutes.

Sauté Onion and Garlic: Add onion and garlic and sauté until fragrant, about 2 minutes.

Add Vegetables: Stir in snap peas, bell peppers, and carrots. Cook for 5-7 minutes, until the veggies are soft and crisp.

Prepare Sauce: Mix soy sauce, rice vinegar, hoisin sauce, sesame oil, and grated ginger in a small bowl.

Combine and Cook: Pour sauce over turkey and vegetables, stirring well to combine. Cook for another 2-3 minutes until heated through and sauce thickens slightly.

Garnish and serve with chopped cilantro.

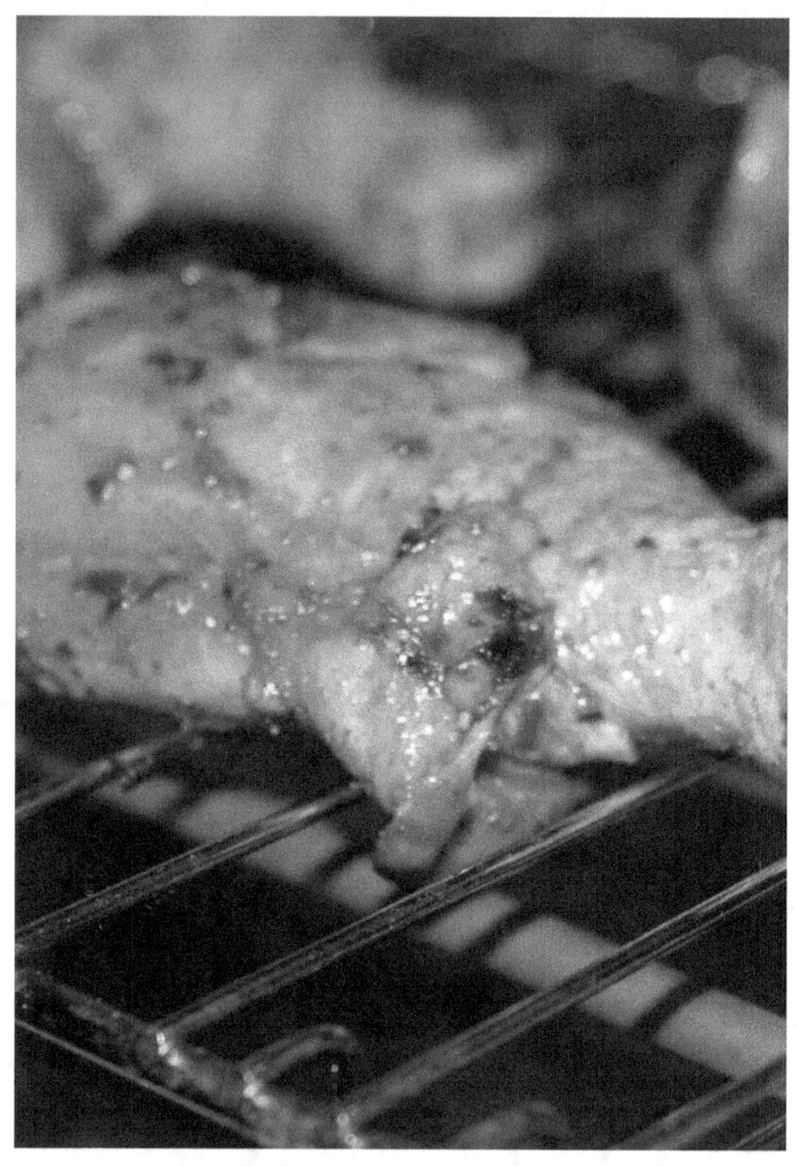

Honey Mustard Glazed Chicken Thighs

Description: Juicy and flavorful chicken thighs with a balanced sweet and tangy honey mustard glaze, perfect for a quick and delicious weeknight dinner.

Cooking Time: 35 minutes

Prep Time: 10 minutes

Servings: 4

Ingredients:

8 boneless, skinless chicken thighs

1/4 cup Dijon mustard

1/4 cup honey

2 tbsp olive oil

1 tbsp apple cider vinegar

2 cloves garlic, minced

1 tsp dried thyme

Salt and pepper to taste

Fresh parsley for garnish

Nutritional Information (per serving):

Calories: 350

Protein: 28g

Fat: 18g

Carbohydrates: 18g

Fiber: 1g

Preparation Steps:

Preheat Oven: Preheat oven to 375°F (190°C). Grease a baking dish.

Prepare Glaze: Whisk together Dijon mustard, honey, olive oil, apple cider vinegar, garlic, thyme, salt, and pepper in a bowl.

Coat Chicken: Place chicken thighs in the baking dish and pour the honey mustard mixture over them, turning to coat evenly.

Bake: Bake for 30-35 minutes or until chicken thighs are cooked through and internal temperature reaches 165°F (74°C).

Garnish and Serve: Garnish with fresh parsley before serving.

CHAPTER 9:

FRESH SEAFOOD

Welcome to the world of fresh seafood! This chapter is dedicated to exploring the flavorful and nutritious world of seafood. With a variety of recipes to choose from, you'll find something to satisfy your cravings and support your digestive health. From delicate baked cod to bold Cajun blackened catfish, our seafood recipes are sure to impress.

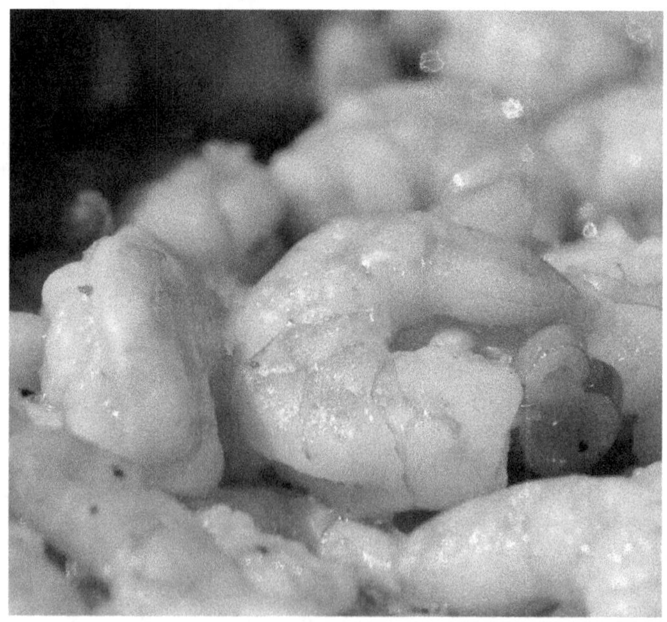

Grilled Lemon Garlic Shrimp

Description: Juicy and tender shrimp infused with a flavorful lemon garlic marinade, perfect for a quick and delicious summer barbecue or weeknight meal.

Cooking Time: 10 minutes

Prep Time: 15 minutes

Servings: 4

Ingredients:

1 lb large shrimp, peeled and deveined

2 tbsp olive oil

3 cloves garlic, minced

Zest of 1 lemon

Juice of 1 lemon

1 tbsp fresh parsley, chopped

Salt and pepper to taste

Lemon wedges for serving

Nutritional Information (per serving):

Calories: 150

Protein: 20g

Fat: 7g

Carbohydrates: 2g

Fiber: 0g

Preparation Steps:

Prepare Marinade: Combine olive oil, garlic, lemon zest, lemon juice, parsley, salt, and pepper in a bowl.

Marinate Shrimp: Add shrimp to the marinade and toss to coat evenly. Let marinate for 10-15 minutes.

Grill Shrimp: Preheat the grill to medium-high heat. Thread shrimp onto skewers and grill for 2-3 minutes per side, until pink and opaque.

Serve hot, with lemon wedges on the side.

Tips and Variations:

Use fresh and sustainable shrimp

Adjust the amount of garlic and lemon to taste

Add other herbs like thyme or rosemary to the marinade

Serve with a side of quinoa or rice and steamed vegetables

Make it a seafood skewer with scallops and bell peppers

Baked Cod with Herbed Crust

Description: A simple yet elegant dish featuring cod fillets topped with a flavorful herbed crust, perfect for special occasions or cozy dinners at home.

Cooking Time: 20 minutes

Prep Time: 10 minutes

Servings: 4

Ingredients:

4 cod filets (6 oz each)

1/4 cup breadcrumbs

2 tbsp grated Parmesan cheese

1 tbsp fresh parsley, chopped

1 tbsp fresh dill, chopped

1 tbsp olive oil

1 clove garlic, minced

Salt and pepper to taste

Lemon wedges for serving

Nutritional Information (per serving):

Calories: 250

Protein: 30g

Fat: 9g

Carbohydrates: 7g

Fiber: 1g

Preparation Steps:

Preheat Oven: Preheat oven to 400°F (200°C). Prepare a baking sheet with parchment paper.

Prepare Herbed Crust: Combine breadcrumbs, Parmesan cheese, parsley, dill, olive oil, garlic, salt, and pepper in a bowl.

Prepare Cod: Place cod fillets on the prepared baking sheet. Pat them dry with paper towels.

Apply Herbed Crust: Spread the breadcrumb mixture evenly over the top of each cod fillet, pressing gently to adhere.

Bake: Bake for 15-20 minutes or until cod is cooked through and flakes easily with a fork.

Serve hot, with lemon wedges on the side.

Tips and Variations:

Use fresh and sustainable cod

Adjust the amount of herbs to taste

Add other herbs like thyme or rosemary to the breadcrumb mixture

Serve with a side of quinoa or roasted vegetables.

Make it a seafood dinner with grilled shrimp or scallops

Pan-seared scallops with Lemon Butter Sauce

Description: Elegant, flavorful, and easy to make, these pan-seared scallops are seared to perfection and topped with a luxurious lemon butter sauce.

Cooking Time: 10 minutes

Prep Time: 5 minutes

Servings: 4

Ingredients:

1 lb large sea scallops, patted dry

Salt and pepper to taste

2 tbsp unsalted butter

2 cloves garlic, minced

Zest of 1 lemon

Juice of 1 lemon

2 tbsp chopped fresh parsley

Lemon wedges for serving

Nutritional Information (per serving):

Calories: 180

Protein: 20g

Fat: 8g

Carbohydrates: 4g

Fiber: 0g

Preparation Steps:

Season Scallops: Season scallops generously with salt and pepper on both sides.

Sear Scallops: Heat a large skillet over medium-high heat. Add butter, then scallops in a single layer. Sear for 2-3 minutes per side, until golden brown and caramelized.

Prepare Lemon Butter Sauce: Remove scallops from the skillet. Add garlic, lemon zest, lemon juice, and parsley to the skillet. Cook for 2 minutes, stirring constantly.

Coat Scallops in Sauce: Return scallops to skillet and toss in lemon butter sauce to coat evenly.

Serving suggestions: Serve hot with lemon wedges on the side.

Tips and Variations:

Use fresh and sustainable scallops

Adjust the amount of lemon and garlic to your liking.

Add other herbs like thyme or rosemary to the lemon butter sauce

Serve with a side of quinoa or roasted vegetables.

Make it a seafood dinner with grilled shrimp or fish

Garlic Butter Salmon

Description: Flavorful and easy to make, this garlic butter salmon is a perfect dish for any occasion. Tender salmon fillets are cooked to perfection in a rich garlic butter sauce.

Cooking Time: 15 minutes

Prep Time: 10 minutes

Servings: 4

Ingredients:

4 salmon filets (6 oz each)

Salt and pepper to taste

2 tbsp unsalted butter

4 cloves garlic, minced

Juice of 1 lemon

2 tbsp chopped fresh parsley

Lemon wedges for serving

Nutritional Information (per serving):

Calories: 320

Protein: 34g

Fat: 18g

Carbohydrates: 2g

Fiber: 0g

Preparation Steps:

Season Salmon: Season salmon fillets with salt and pepper on both sides.

Prepare Garlic Butter: Melt butter in a large skillet over medium heat. Add garlic and cook for 1 minute until fragrant.

Cook Salmon: Add salmon fillets to skillet, skin-side down. Cook for 4-5 minutes until golden brown. Flip and cook for another 4-5 minutes until cooked through.

Finish with Lemon and Parsley: Remove from heat. Squeeze lemon juice over salmon and sprinkle with parsley.

Serve hot, with lemon wedges on the side.

Tips and Variations:

Use fresh and sustainable salmon

Adjust the amount of garlic and lemon to taste

Add other herbs like thyme or rosemary to the garlic butter sauce

Serve with a side of quinoa or roasted vegetables.

Make it a seafood dinner with grilled shrimp or scallops

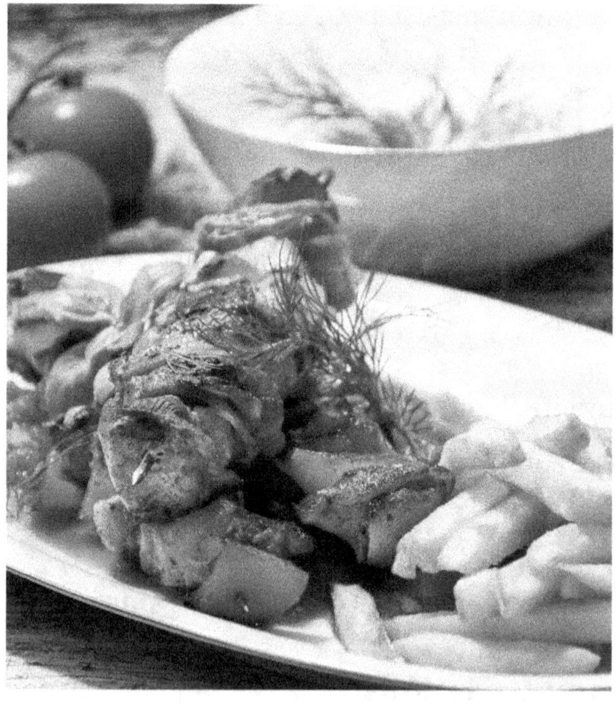

Coconut Curry Shrimp

Description: A flavorful and aromatic dish, coconut curry shrimp combines succulent shrimp with creamy coconut milk and fragrant spices. Quick and easy to prepare, ideal for a midweek dinner.

Cooking Time: 20 minutes

Prep Time: 10 minutes

Servings: 4

Ingredients:

1 lb large shrimp, peeled and deveined

2 tbsp coconut oil

1 onion, finely chopped

3 cloves garlic, minced

1 tbsp grated ginger

2 tbsp red curry paste

1 can (14 oz) coconut milk

1 red bell pepper, sliced

1 green bell pepper, sliced

1 cup snap peas

Salt and pepper to taste

Fresh cilantro for garnish

Cooked rice for serving

Nutritional Information (per serving, without rice):

Calories: 250

Protein: 20g

Fat: 18g

Carbohydrates: 8g

Fiber: 2g

Preparation Steps:

Sauté Aromatics: Heat coconut oil in a large skillet over medium heat. Add onion, garlic, and ginger. Sauté until fragrant, about 2 minutes.

Add Curry Paste: Stir in red curry paste and cook for another minute.

Add Coconut Milk and Vegetables: Add coconut milk, bell peppers, and snap peas to the skillet. Cook for 5-7 minutes, until the veggies are soft and crisp.

Add Shrimp: Add shrimp to the skillet and cook for 3-4 minutes until pink and opaque.

Season and serve with salt and pepper to taste. Garnish with fresh cilantro. Serve hot cooked rice.

Tips and Variations:

Use fresh and sustainable shrimp

Adjust the amount of curry paste to the desired spice level

Add other vegetables like carrots or potatoes

Serve with naan bread or roti for a different twist

Make it a seafood dinner with grilled fish or scallops

Citrus Herb Baked Tilapia

Description: A light and flavorful dish, this citrus herb-baked tilapia is a healthy dinner option. Tilapia fillets are marinated in a zesty citrus herb mixture and baked to perfection, resulting in tender and flaky fish packed with flavor.

Cooking Time: 20 minutes

Prep Time: 10 minutes

Servings: 4

Ingredients:

4 tilapia fillets (about 6 oz each)

Zest and juice of 1 lemon

Zest and juice of 1 lime

2 tbsp olive oil

2 cloves garlic, minced

1 tbsp chopped fresh parsley

1 tbsp chopped fresh dill

Salt and pepper to taste

Lemon and lime wedges for serving

Nutritional Information (per serving):

Calories: 200

Protein: 25g

Fat: 9g

Carbohydrates: 2g

Fiber: 0g

Preparation Steps:

Preheat Oven: Preheat oven to 400°F (200°C). Prepare a baking sheet with parchment paper.

Prepare Citrus Herb Mixture: Whisk together lemon zest, lemon juice, lime zest, lime juice, olive oil, garlic, parsley, dill, salt, and pepper in a bowl.

Marinate Tilapia: Place tilapia fillets on the prepared baking sheet. Pour the citrus herb mixture over the tilapia, ensuring an even coating.

Bake: Bake for 15-20 minutes or until tilapia is cooked through and flakes easily with a fork.

Serve: Serve hot with lemon and lime wedges on the side.

Tips and Variations:

Use fresh and sustainable tilapia

Adjust the amount of citrus and herbs to taste

Add other herbs like thyme or rosemary to the citrus herb mixture

Serve with a side of quinoa or roasted vegetables.

Make it a seafood dinner with grilled shrimp or scallops

Cajun Blackened Catfish

Description: A spicy and flavorful dish, this Cajun blackened catfish is perfect for a Southern-inspired meal. Catfish fillets are coated in a bold blend of Cajun spices and seared to perfection, resulting in a crispy exterior and tender, flaky fish.

Cooking Time: 15 minutes

Prep Time: 10 minutes

Servings: 4

Ingredients:

4 catfish filets (about 6 oz each)

2 tbsp Cajun seasoning

2 tbsp olive oil

Lemon wedges for serving

Nutritional Information (per serving):

Calories: 280

Protein: 25g

Fat: 14g

Carbohydrates: 2g

Fiber: 1g

Preparation Steps:

Season Catfish: Rub Cajun seasoning evenly on both sides of catfish filets.

Heat the olive oil in a large skillet over medium-high heat.

Cook Catfish: Add catfish filets to the skillet. Cook for 3-4 minutes per side, or until the salmon is browned and well cooked.

Serve: Remove catfish from skillet and serve hot with lemon wedges on the side.

Tips and Variations:

Use fresh and sustainable catfish

Adjust the amount of Cajun seasoning to the desired spice level

Add other spices like paprika or garlic powder to the Cajun seasoning blend

Serve with a side of hushpuppies or coleslaw

Make it a seafood dinner with grilled shrimp or scallops

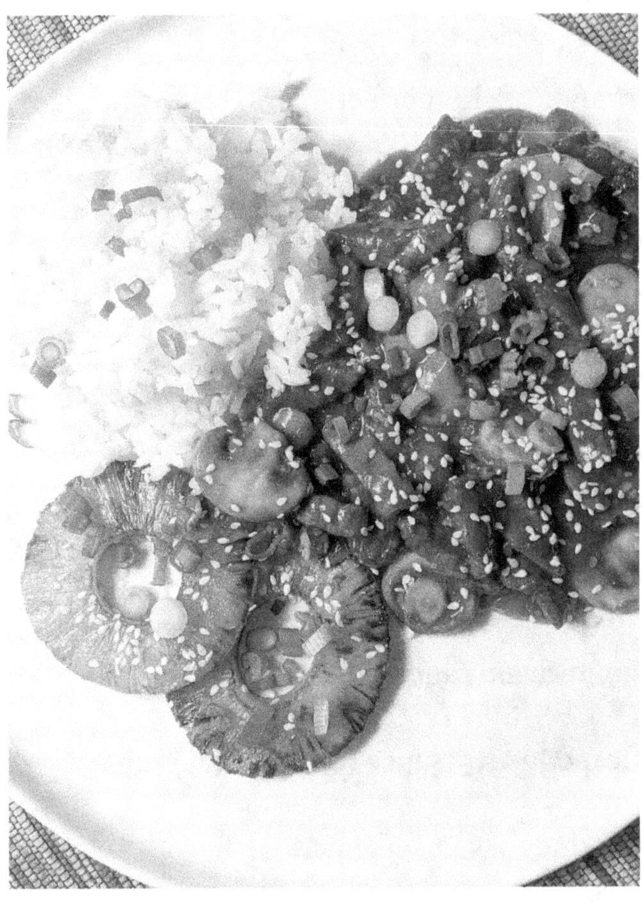

Teriyaki Glazed Mahi Mahi

Description: A delightful dish combining the sweetness of teriyaki sauce with the succulence of mahi mahi fish, perfectly grilled to indulge your senses and taste buds.

Cooking Time: 15 minutes

Prep Time: 10 minutes

Servings: 4

Ingredients:

4 mahi mahi fillets (6 oz each)

1/4 cup teriyaki sauce

2 tablespoons soy sauce (or tamari if gluten-free)

2 tbsp honey

1 tbsp rice vinegar

2 cloves garlic, minced

1 tsp grated ginger

1 tbsp sesame seeds

Sliced green onions for garnish

Nutritional Information (per serving):

Calories: 280

Protein: 34g

Fat: 8g

Carbohydrates: 14g

Fiber: 1g

Preparation Steps:

Prepare Teriyaki Marinade: Whisk together teriyaki sauce, soy sauce, honey, rice vinegar, garlic, and ginger in a bowl.

Marinate Mahi Mahi: Place mahi mahi filets in a shallow dish or resealable plastic bag. Pour teriyaki marinade over filets, coating well. Marinate in the refrigerator for a minimum of 30 minutes.

Grill Mahi Mahi: Preheat the grill to medium-high heat. Remove filets from the marinade, discarding excess. Grill for 4-5 minutes per side, or until cooked through and opaque.

Glaze and Serve: Brush remaining teriyaki marinade over grilled mahi mahi. Sprinkle sesame seeds and sliced green onions over filets before serving.

Tips and Variations:

Use fresh and sustainable mahi mahi

Adjust the teriyaki sauce amount to the desired sweetness level

Add other ingredients like pineapple or bell peppers to the teriyaki marinade

Serve with a side of steamed vegetables or Japanese rice

Make it a seafood dinner with grilled shrimp or scallops

Mediterranean Style Grilled Swordfish

Description: Transport yourself to the Mediterranean shores with this grilled swordfish dish, seasoned with a blend of Mediterranean herbs and spices. Juicy and flavorful, this dish celebrates fresh ingredients and bold flavors.

Cooking Time: 15 minutes

Prep Time: 10 minutes

Servings: 4

Ingredients:

4 swordfish steaks (6 oz each)

2 tbsp olive oil

2 cloves garlic, minced

Zest and juice of 1 lemon

1 tbsp chopped fresh oregano

1 tbsp chopped fresh parsley

1 tsp dried thyme

Salt and pepper to taste

Lemon wedges for serving

Nutritional Information (per serving):

Calories: 320

Protein: 30g

Fat: 18g

Carbohydrates: 3g

Fiber: 1g

Preparation Steps:

Prepare Mediterranean Marinade: Whisk together olive oil, garlic, lemon zest, lemon juice, oregano, parsley, thyme, salt, and pepper in a bowl.

Marinate Swordfish: Place swordfish steaks in a shallow dish or resealable plastic bag. Pour Mediterranean marinade over steaks, coating well. Marinate in the refrigerator for a minimum of 30 minutes.

Grill Swordfish: Preheat the grill to medium-high heat. Remove swordfish steaks from marinade, discarding excess. Grill for 5-6 minutes per side, or until cooked through and flaky.

Serve hot, with lemon wedges on the side.

Tips and Variations:

Use fresh and sustainable swordfish

Adjust the amount of garlic and herbs to taste

Add other Mediterranean ingredients like feta cheese or olives to the marinade

Serve with a side of grilled vegetables or quinoa

Make it a seafood dinner with grilled shrimp or scallops

CHAPTER 10:

CRISP SALADS AND SIDES

Brighten up your meals with a rainbow of fresh salads and sides! This chapter presents a vibrant collection of crisp and colorful dishes that perfectly complement any main course. Indulge in the classic Greek salad, refreshing watermelon feta salad, and more nutrient-packed recipes that burst with flavor.

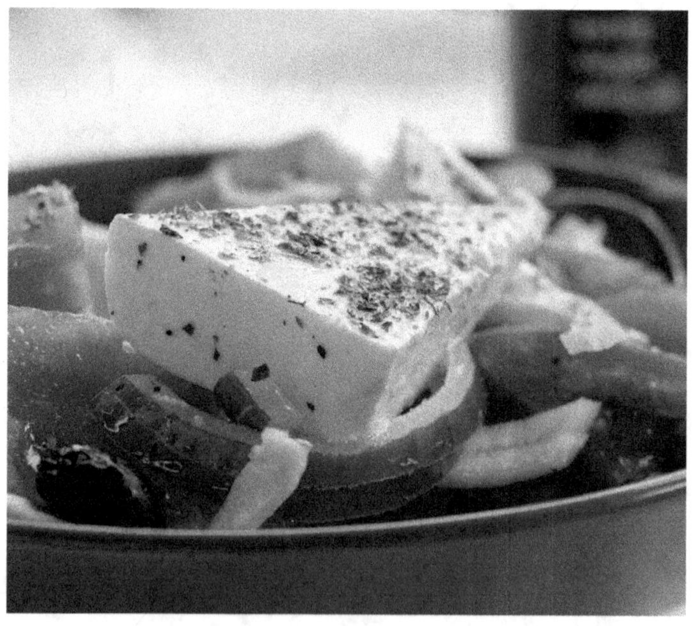

Greek Salad with Feta and Olives

Description: Enjoy the flavors of the Mediterranean with this classic Greek salad, featuring crisp lettuce, juicy tomatoes, crunchy cucumbers, tangy feta cheese, and briny olives, all tossed in a light and refreshing vinaigrette.

Prep Time: 15 minutes

Servings: 4

Ingredients:

4 cups mixed salad greens

1 cup cherry tomatoes, halved

1 cucumber, sliced

1/2 red onion, thinly sliced

1/2 cup Kalamata olives, pitted

1/2 cup crumbled feta cheese

2 tbsp extra virgin olive oil

1 tbsp red wine vinegar

1 tsp dried oregano

Salt and pepper to taste

Nutritional Information (per serving):

Calories: 180

Protein: 5g

Fat: 14g

Carbohydrates: 10g

Fiber: 3g

Preparation Steps:

Combine Salad Ingredients: In a large salad bowl, combine mixed salad greens, cherry tomatoes, cucumber slices, red onion slices, Kalamata olives, and crumbled feta cheese.

Make Dressing: Whisk together olive oil, red wine vinegar, dried oregano, salt, and pepper to make the dressing.

Toss Salad: Add the dressing to the salad and toss gently to combine.

Serve: Serve immediately as a refreshing side dish or a light and satisfying meal on its own.

Tips and Variations:

Customize with your favorite ingredients or proteins like grilled chicken or salmon

Add a sprinkle of crumbled feta cheese for extra flavor

Use different types of olives or cheese for a unique twist

Make ahead and store in the refrigerator for a quick and easy meal prep

Cobb Salad with Avocado and Bacon

Description: Enjoy a hearty and satisfying meal with this classic Cobb salad, featuring crisp lettuce, diced avocado, crispy bacon, juicy cherry tomatoes, tender grilled chicken breast, hard-boiled eggs, and crumbled blue cheese, sprinkled with a zesty vinaigrette.

Prep Time: 20 minutes

Cooking Time: 20 minutes

Servings: 4

Ingredients:

6 cups mixed salad greens

2 boneless, skinless chicken breasts

4 slices bacon, cooked and crumbled

2 hard-boiled eggs, sliced

1 avocado, diced

1 cup cherry tomatoes, halved

1/4 cup crumbled blue cheese

2 tbsp extra virgin olive oil

1 tbsp red wine vinegar

1 tsp Dijon mustard

Salt and pepper to taste

Nutritional Information (per serving):

Calories: 350

Protein: 25g

Fat: 24g

Carbohydrates: 10g

Fiber: 5g

Preparation Steps:

Grill Chicken: Season chicken breasts with salt and pepper. Grill or pan-sear until cooked through, about 6-8 minutes per side. Let sit for 5 minutes before slicing into strips.

Assemble Salad: Arrange mixed salad greens in a large bowl. Add rows of sliced grilled chicken, crumbled bacon, hard-boiled egg slices, diced avocado, cherry tomato halves, and crumbled blue cheese.

Make Dressing: Whisk together olive oil, red wine vinegar, Dijon mustard, salt, and pepper in a small bowl.

Drizzle Dressing: Drizzle dressing over the Cobb salad or serve on the side. Toss gently to coat or serve as a deconstructed salad.

Tips and Variations:

Customize with your favorite ingredients or proteins like salmon or tofu

Add a sprinkle of crumbled blue cheese for extra flavor

Use different types of cheese or nuts for a unique twist

Make ahead and store in the refrigerator for a quick and easy meal prep

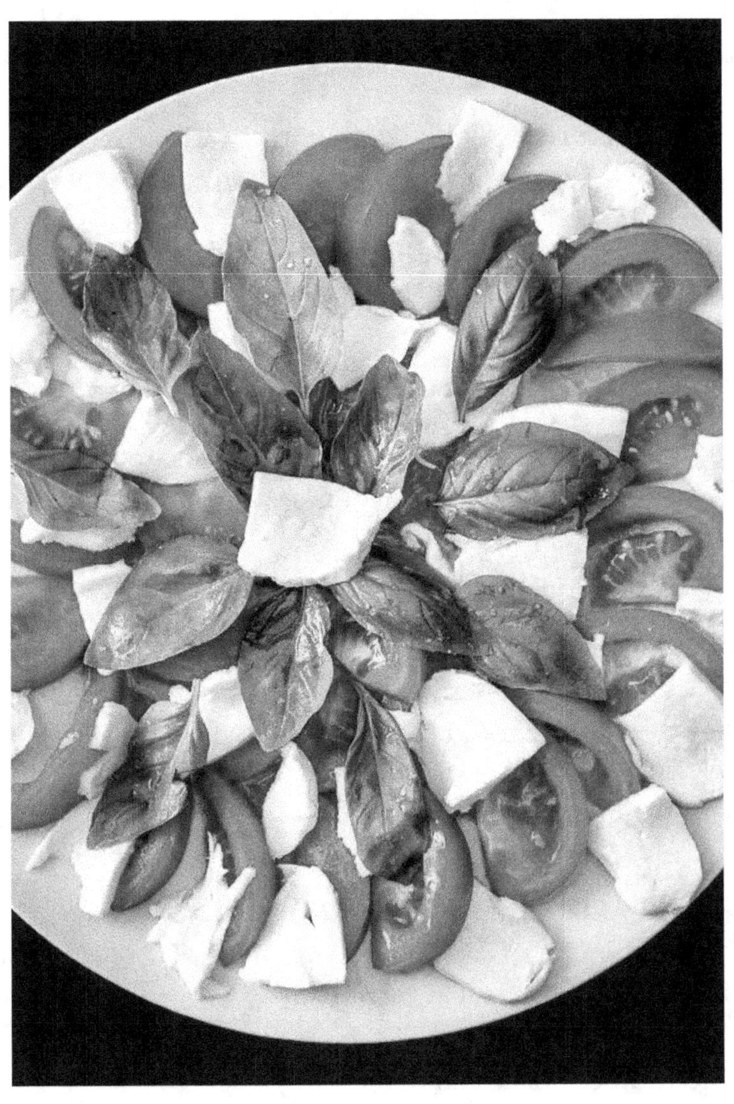

Caprese Salad with Balsamic Glaze

Description: Enjoy the flavors of Italy with this elegant Caprese salad, featuring layers of ripe tomatoes, fresh mozzarella cheese, and fragrant basil leaves, all drizzled with a tangy balsamic glaze.

Prep Time: 10 minutes

Servings: 4

Ingredients:

2 large ripe tomatoes, sliced

8 oz fresh mozzarella cheese, sliced

Fresh basil leaves

Balsamic glaze (store-bought or homemade)

Extra virgin olive oil

Salt and pepper to taste

Nutritional Information (per serving):

Calories: 220

Protein: 14g

Fat: 15g

Carbohydrates: 8g

Fiber: 2g

Preparation Steps:

Arrange Salad: Alternate sliced tomatoes and mozzarella cheese on a serving platter.

Add Fresh Basil: Tuck basil leaves between tomato and mozzarella slices.

Drizzle Dressing: Drizzle balsamic glaze and extra virgin olive oil over the salad.

Season with salt and pepper, to taste.

Serve: Serve immediately as a light and refreshing appetizer or side dish.

Tips and Variations:

Use heirloom tomatoes for a colorful twist

Add a sprinkle of Parmesan cheese for extra flavor

Substitute burrata cheese for a creamy surprise

Make ahead and store in the refrigerator for up to 2 hours

Serve as a light lunch or dinner accompaniment

Asian Cucumber Salad

Description: Enjoy the vibrant flavors of Asia with this refreshing cucumber salad, featuring thinly sliced cucumbers tossed in a tangy dressing made with rice vinegar, soy sauce, sesame oil, and a hint of sweetness.

Prep Time: 10 minutes

Servings: 4

Ingredients:

2 large cucumbers, thinly sliced

2 tbsp rice vinegar

1 tablespoon soy sauce (or tamari if gluten-free)

1 tsp sesame oil

1 tsp sugar (or sweetener of choice)

1 clove garlic, minced

1 tsp sesame seeds

Thinly sliced green onions for garnish

Nutritional Information (per serving):

Calories: 40

Protein: 1g

Fat: 2g

Carbohydrates: 6g

Fiber: 1g

Preparation Steps:

Make Dressing: Whisk together rice vinegar, soy sauce, sesame oil, sugar, and garlic in a small bowl.

Toss Cucumbers: Place sliced cucumbers in a serving bowl and pour dressing over them. Toss gently to coat.

Garnish: Sprinkle sesame seeds and green onions over the cucumber salad.

Serve: Serve immediately as a refreshing side dish or light and healthy snack.

Tips and Variations:

Add diced bell peppers or carrots for extra crunch

Substitute honey or maple syrup for sugar

Use gluten-free soy sauce or tamari as a gluten-free option.

Make ahead and store in the refrigerator for up to 2 hours

Serve as a side dish or add to noodle or rice bowls for a flavorful topping

Spinach Strawberry Salad with Balsamic Vinaigrette

Description: A refreshing salad bursting with flavors, perfect for a light lunch or side dish.

Cooking Time: 10 minutes

Prep Time: 15 minutes

Servings: 4

Ingredients:

6 cups fresh baby spinach

1 cup sliced strawberries

1/4 cup chopped walnuts

2 tablespoons balsamic vinegar

1 tablespoon extra virgin olive oil

1 teaspoon honey

Salt and pepper to taste

Nutritional Information (per serving):

Calories: 120

Total Fat: 8g

Carbohydrates: 10g

Fiber: 3g

Protein: 3g

Preparation Steps:

Combine Salad Ingredients: In a large bowl, combine spinach, strawberries, and walnuts.

Make Vinaigrette: Whisk together balsamic vinegar, olive oil, honey, salt, and pepper in a small bowl.

Dress the Salad: Pour vinaigrette over the salad and toss gently to coat.

Serve: Serve immediately and enjoy the flavor burst!

Tips and Variations:

Add crumbled feta cheese for extra flavor

Substitute almonds or pecans for walnuts

Use different types of vinegar or sweetener to change the flavor profile

Make ahead and store in the refrigerator for up to 2 hours

Serve as a light lunch or as a side dish for your favorite meals

Quinoa Salad with Roasted Vegetables

Description: A hearty salad packed with protein and nutrients, perfect for a satisfying meal.

Cooking Time: 25 minutes

Prep Time: 15 minutes

Servings: 4

Ingredients:

1 cup quinoa, rinsed

2 cups water

2 cups mixed vegetables (such as bell peppers, zucchini, and cherry tomatoes), chopped

2 tablespoons olive oil

1 teaspoon dried herbs (such as thyme or rosemary)

Salt and pepper to taste

Juice of 1 lemon

Nutritional Information (per serving):

Calories: 240

Total Fat: 8g

Carbohydrates: 36g

Fiber: 6g

Protein: 8g

Preparation Steps:

Cook Quinoa: Preheat the oven to 400°F (200°C). In a medium saucepan, mix the quinoa and water.

Bring to a boil, then reduce heat and simmer for 15 minutes or until quinoa is tender and water is absorbed.

Roast Vegetables: On a baking sheet, toss mixed vegetables with olive oil, dried herbs, salt, and pepper. Roast in a warm oven for 20-25 minutes, until soft and caramelized.

Combine Quinoa and Vegetables: In a large bowl, combine cooked quinoa and roasted vegetables. Squeeze lemon juice over the salad and toss gently to combine.

Serve: Serve warm or at room temperature for a delightful meal.

Tips and Variations:

Add protein sources like grilled chicken, salmon, or tofu for added flavor and nutrition

Mix in other vegetables like sweet potatoes, Brussels sprouts, or broccoli

Change the flavor profile by adding different herbs and spices.

Make ahead and store in the refrigerator for up to 3 days

Serve as a main dish or as a side for your favorite meals

Kale Caesar Salad with Parmesan Crisps

Description: A modern twist on a classic Caesar salad, featuring hearty kale and crispy Parmesan crisps. Cooking Time: 15 minutes

Prep Time: 10 minutes

Servings: 4

Ingredients:

1 bunch kale, stems removed, leaves torn into bite-sized pieces.

½ cup grated Parmesan cheese

2 tablespoons olive oil

2 tablespoons lemon juice

1 teaspoon Dijon mustard

1 garlic clove, minced

Salt and pepper to taste

Nutritional Information (per serving):

Calories: 180

Total Fat: 12g Carbohydrates: 12g Fiber: 3g

Protein: 8g

Preparation Steps:

Preheat the oven to 375°F (190°C).

On a baking sheet lined with parchment paper, form 4 piles of grated Parmesan cheese, spreading each pile into a thin layer. Bake the Parmesan crisps in the preheated oven for 5-7 minutes, or until golden and crispy. Remove from the oven and allow to cool.

In a large bowl, massage the kale leaves with olive oil for a few minutes to soften them.

In a small bowl, whisk together the lemon juice, Dijon mustard, minced garlic, salt, and pepper to create the Caesar dressing. Pour the dressing over the kale and toss gently to coat. Crumble the

Parmesan crisps over the salad just before serving for a satisfying crunch.

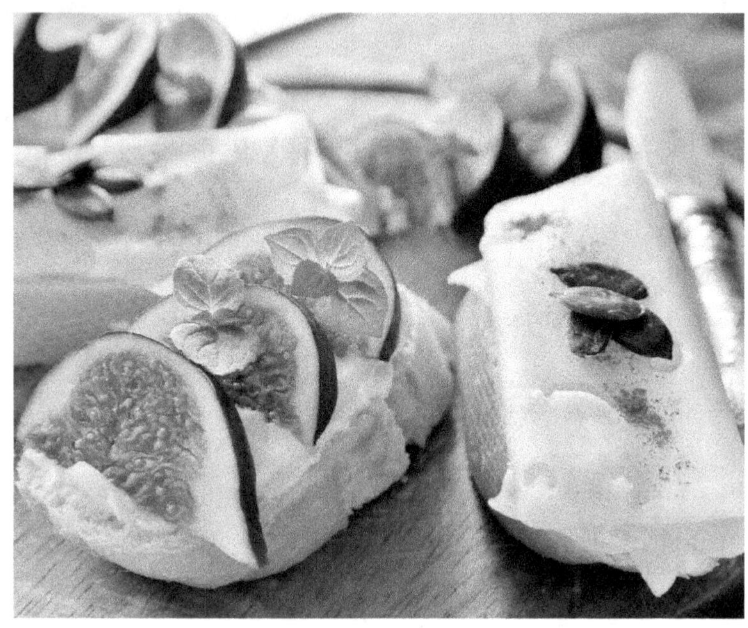

Beet and Goat Cheese Salad with Walnuts

Description: A vibrant salad featuring earthy beets, creamy goat cheese, and crunchy walnuts, perfect for any occasion.

Cooking Time: 45 minutes

Prep Time: 20 minutes

Servings: 4

Ingredients:

4 medium beets, roasted, peeled, and sliced

2 cups mixed salad greens

1/2 cup crumbled goat cheese

1/4 cup chopped walnuts

2 tablespoons balsamic vinegar

1 tablespoon honey

2 tablespoons extra virgin olive oil

Salt and pepper to taste

Nutritional Information (per serving):

Calories: 220

Total Fat: 14g

Carbohydrates: 20g

Fiber: 4g

Protein: 6g

Preparation Steps:

Roast Beets: Preheat oven to 400°F (200°C). Wrap each beet in aluminum foil and roast for 45-60 minutes, or until tender. Let cool, then peel and slice.

Assemble Salad: In a large bowl, combine roasted beet slices, mixed salad greens, crumbled goat cheese, and chopped walnuts.

Make Vinaigrette: Whisk together balsamic vinegar, honey, olive oil, salt, and pepper in a small bowl.

Dress Salad: Drizzle vinaigrette over the salad and toss gently to coat.

Serve: Serve immediately and enjoy the harmonious blend of flavors and textures.

Tips and Variations:

Add grilled chicken or salmon for added protein

Substitute feta cheese for goat cheese

Use different types of nuts or seeds for added crunch

Make ahead and store in the refrigerator for up to 2 hours

Serve as a main dish or as a side for your favorite meals

Watermelon Feta Salad with Mint

Description: A refreshing and summery salad that combines the sweetness of watermelon with the tanginess of feta cheese and the freshness of mint.

Cooking Time: 15 minutes

Prep Time: 10 minutes

Servings: 4

Ingredients:

4 cups cubed seedless watermelon

1 cup crumbled feta cheese

1/4 cup fresh mint leaves, chopped

2 tablespoons extra virgin olive oil

1 tablespoon balsamic vinegar

Salt and pepper to taste

Nutritional Information (per serving):

Calories: 180

Total Fat: 12g

Carbohydrates: 15g

Fiber: 1g

Protein: 6g

Preparation Steps:

Combine Salad Ingredients: In a large bowl, combine cubed watermelon, crumbled feta cheese, and chopped mint leaves.

Drizzle Dressing: Drizzle olive oil and balsamic vinegar over the salad. Add salt and pepper to taste.

Toss Salad: Gently toss the salad to combine all the ingredients.

Serve: Serve chilled and enjoy the delightful contrast of flavors and textures.

Tips and Variations:

Add grilled chicken or prawns for extra protein.

Substitute goat cheese for feta cheese

Use different types of mint or herbs for a unique flavor

Make ahead and store in the refrigerator for up to 2 hours

Serve as a light and refreshing side dish or as a main course for a summer meal.

Southwest Black Bean and Corn Salad

Description: A vibrant and flavorful salad inspired by the bold flavors of the Southwest, featuring black beans, corn, tomatoes, avocado, and a zesty lime dressing.

Cooking Time: 10 minutes

Prep Time: 15 minutes

Servings: 4

Ingredients:

1 can (15 ounces) of black beans, washed and drained

1 cup corn kernels (fresh, frozen, or canned)

1 cup cherry tomatoes, halved

1 avocado, diced

1/4 cup red onion, finely chopped

1/4 cup fresh cilantro, chopped

Juice of 2 limes

2 tablespoons extra virgin olive oil

1 teaspoon ground cumin

Salt and pepper to taste

Nutritional Information (per serving):

Calories: 250

Total Fat: 12g

Carbohydrates: 30g

Fiber: 10g

Protein: 8g

Preparation Steps:

Combine Salad Ingredients: In a large bowl, combine black beans, corn kernels, cherry tomatoes, diced avocado, chopped red onion, and chopped cilantro.

Make Dressing: Whisk together lime juice, olive oil, ground cumin, salt, and pepper in a small bowl.

Dress Salad: Pour dressing over salad ingredients and gently toss to coat.

Serve: Serve immediately or refrigerate for later, allowing flavors to meld together.

Tips and Variations:

Add diced grilled chicken or shrimp for extra protein

Use different types of beans or corn for variation

Add diced bell peppers or jalapeños for added flavor.

Make ahead and refrigerate for up to 24 hours.

Serve as a main dish or as a side for your favorite meals.

CHAPTER 11:

DESSERTS

Indulge in guilt-free treats that satisfy your sweet tooth without compromising your digestive health. This chapter presents decadent and refreshing desserts, carefully crafted to delight your taste buds while prioritizing wellness.

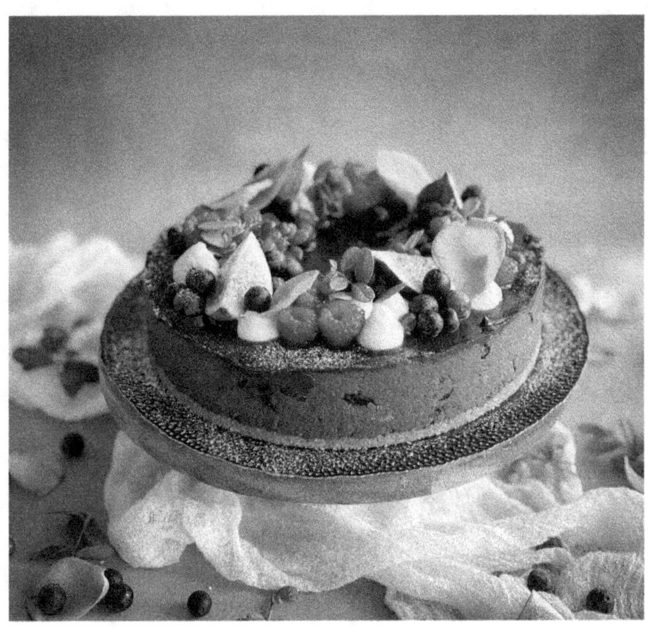

Flourless Chocolate Cake

Description: Indulge guilt-free in this decadent flourless chocolate cake that's rich, moist, and incredibly satisfying, suitable for any occasion.

Cooking Time: 30 minutes

Prep Time: 15 minutes

Servings: 8

Ingredients:

1 cup semisweet chocolate chips

1/2 cup unsalted butter

3/4 cup granulated sugar

3 large eggs

1 teaspoon vanilla extract

Pinch of salt

Fresh berries for garnish (optional)

Powdered sugar for dusting (optional)

Nutritional Information (per serving):

Calories: 320

Total Fat: 20g

Carbohydrates: 30g

Fiber: 2g

Protein: 4g

Preparation Steps:

Preheat and Prep Pan: Preheat oven to 350°F(175°C). Grease a 9-inch round cake pan and line its bottom with parchment paper.

Melt Chocolate and Butter: In a heatproof bowl set over a pot of simmering water, melt chocolate chips and butter together, stirring until smooth. Remove from heat and allow it to cool slightly.

Whisk Egg Mixture: In a separate bowl, whisk together sugar, eggs, vanilla extract, and salt until well combined.

Combine Chocolate and Egg Mixtures: Pour melted chocolate mixture into egg mixture, stirring until smooth and glossy.

Pour into Prepared Pan: Pour batter into prepared cake pan and smooth the top with a spatula.

Bake: Bake in a preheated oven for 25-30 minutes, or until the edges are set but the center is still soft.

Cool and Garnish: Remove from the oven and let cool in the pan for 10 minutes before transferring to a wire rack to cool completely. Garnish with fresh berries and dust with powdered sugar if desired.

Serve and Enjoy: Slice and serve this indulgent flourless chocolate cake, and savor every rich and chocolatey bite!

Greek Yogurt Berry Parfait

Description: A light and refreshing parfait that combines creamy Greek yogurt with sweet berries and crunchy granola, perfect for a healthy dessert or breakfast treat.

Prep Time: 10 minutes

Servings: 2

Ingredients:

1 cup Greek yogurt

1 cup mixed berries (including strawberries, blueberries, and raspberries)

1/2 cup granola

Honey or maple syrup for drizzling (optional)

Nutritional Information (per serving):

Calories: 250

Total Fat: 7g

Carbohydrates: 35g

Fiber: 5g

Protein: 15g

Preparation Steps:

Layer Ingredients: In two serving glasses or bowls, layer Greek yogurt, mixed berries, and granola, repeating until the glasses are filled.

Add Sweetener (Optional): Drizzle honey or maple syrup over the top for added sweetness.

Serve and Enjoy: Serve immediately and enjoy this delightful parfait that's delicious and nutritious!

Almond Flour Banana Bread

Description: A wholesome and moist banana bread made with almond flour, ripe bananas, and a hint of cinnamon, perfect for a guilt-free indulgence any time of day.

Cooking Time: 50 minutes

Prep Time: 15 minutes

Servings: 10

Ingredients:

2 cups almond flour

1 teaspoon baking powder

1/2 teaspoon baking soda

1/2 teaspoon ground cinnamon

Pinch of salt

3 ripe bananas, mashed

3 large eggs

1/4 cup honey or maple syrup

1/4 cup unsalted butter, melted

1 teaspoon vanilla extract

Nutritional Information (per serving):

Calories: 230

Total Fat: 16g

Carbohydrates: 20g

Fiber: 4g

Protein: 7g

Preparation Steps:

Preheat and Prep Pan: Preheat oven to 350°F(175°C). Grease a 9-by-5-inch loaf pan with butter or cooking spray.

Whisk Dry Ingredients: In a large bowl, whisk together almond flour, baking powder, baking soda, cinnamon, and salt.

Mix Wet Ingredients: In a separate bowl, mash ripe bananas, then add eggs, honey or maple syrup, melted butter, and vanilla extract. Mix until well combined.

Combine Wet and Dry Ingredients: Gradually add wet ingredients to dry ingredients, stirring until combined.

Pour into Loaf Pan: Pour batter into the prepared loaf pan and smooth the top with a spatula.

Bake: Bake in a preheated oven for 45-50 minutes, or until a toothpick inserted into the center comes out clean.

Cool and Serve: Remove from the oven and let cool in the pan for 10 minutes before transferring to a wire rack to cool completely. Slice and serve!

Dark Chocolate Avocado Mousse

Description: Indulge in a guilt-free dessert that combines dark chocolate flavors with avocado creaminess.

Cooking Time: 0 minutes

Prep Time: 10 minutes

Servings: 4

Ingredients:

2 ripe avocados

1/4 cup cocoa powder

1/4 cup maple syrup

1 teaspoon vanilla extract

Pinch of salt

Fresh berries for garnish (optional)

Nutritional Information (per serving):

Calories: 180

Total Fat: 12g

Saturated Fat: 2g

Sodium: 5mg

Total Carbohydrates: 18g

Dietary Fiber: 7g

Sugars: 9g

Protein: 2g

Preparation Steps:

Scoop Avocado Flesh: Cut avocados in half, remove pits, and scoop flesh into a blender or food processor.

Add Ingredients: Add cocoa powder, maple syrup, vanilla extract, and a pinch of salt to the blender.

Blend: Blend until smooth and creamy, scraping down sides as needed.

Chill: Transfer mousse to serving bowls and chill in the refrigerator for at least 30 minutes.

Garnish and Serve: Garnish with fresh berries before serving, if desired.

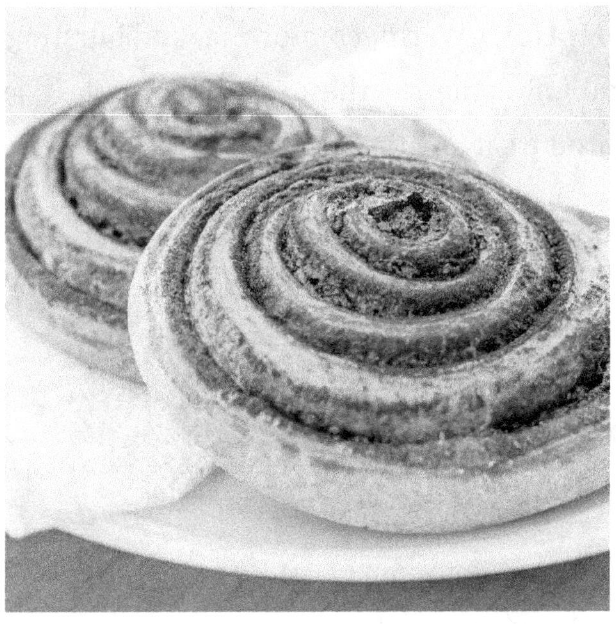

Baked Apples with Cinnamon and Walnuts

Description: Warm, comforting, and bursting with natural sweetness, these baked apples are a delightful treat any time of day.

Cooking Time: 40 minutes

Prep Time: 10 minutes

Servings: 4

Ingredients:

4 large apples (Granny Smith or Honeycrisp)

1/4 cup chopped walnuts

2 tablespoons maple syrup

1 teaspoon ground cinnamon

Pinch of nutmeg (optional)

Nutritional Information (per serving):

Calories: 160

Total Fat: 5g

Saturated Fat: 0.5g

Sodium: 0mg

Total Carbohydrates: 30g

Dietary Fiber: 5g

Sugars: 22g

Protein: 1g

Preparation Steps:

Preheat the oven to 375°F (190°C).

Core Apples: Core the apples, leaving the bottoms intact to create a well for the filling.

Prepare Walnut Mixture: In a small bowl, mix chopped walnuts, maple syrup, cinnamon, and nutmeg (if using).

Stuff Apples: Stuff each apple with the walnut mixture, packing it lightly.

Bake: Place the stuffed apples in a baking dish and bake for 35-40 minutes, or until tender.

Serve: Serve warm, optionally topped with a dollop of yogurt or a drizzle of honey.

Coconut Macaroons

Description: These chewy and sweet coconut macaroons are a delightful treat that's easy to make and perfect for satisfying your sweet tooth.

Cooking Time: 20 minutes

Prep Time: 10 minutes

Servings: 12

Ingredients:

3 cups shredded coconut (unsweetened)

2/3 cup sweetened condensed milk

1 teaspoon vanilla extract

Pinch of salt

Optional: Dark chocolate for dipping

Nutritional Information (per serving):

Calories: 180

Total Fat: 10g

Saturated Fat: 9g

Sodium: 70mg

Total Carbohydrates: 20g

Dietary Fiber: 2g

Sugars: 18g

Protein: 2g

Preparation Steps:

Preheat Oven: Preheat your oven to 325°F (160°C) and line a baking sheet with parchment paper.

Mix Coconut Mixture: In a large bowl, mix shredded coconut, sweetened condensed milk, vanilla extract, and a pinch of salt until well combined.

Form Macaroons: Using a spoon or cookie scoop, form the mixture into small mounds and place them on the prepared baking sheet.

Bake: Bake for 15-20 minutes, or until the macaroons are golden brown around the edges.

Cool: Allow the macaroons to cool completely on the baking sheet before serving.

Dip in Chocolate (Optional): For extra indulgence, melt some dark chocolate and dip the bottoms of the macaroons before setting.

Pumpkin Pie Bites

Description: Enjoy fall flavors with these bite-sized pumpkin pie treats, just right for satisfying your pumpkin spice cravings without guilt.

Cooking Time: 30 minutes

Prep Time: 15 minutes

Servings: 12

Ingredients:

1 cup pumpkin puree

1/4 cup coconut sugar

1 teaspoon pumpkin pie spice

1/2 teaspoon vanilla extract

12 mini phyllo dough shells

Nutritional Information (per serving):

Calories: 70

Total Fat: 2g

Saturated Fat: 1g

Sodium: 35mg

Total Carbohydrates: 12g

Dietary Fiber: 1g

Sugars: 5g

Protein: 1g

Preparation Steps:

Preheat the oven to 350°F (175°C), and prepare a baking sheet with parchment paper.

Mix Pumpkin Mixture: In a bowl, mix pumpkin puree, coconut sugar, pumpkin pie spice, and vanilla extract until well combined.

Fill Phyllo Shells: Spoon the pumpkin mixture into the mini Phyllo dough shells, filling each almost to the top.

Bake: Place the filled shells on the prepared baking sheet and bake for 15-20 minutes, or until the filling is set.

Cool and Serve: Allow the pumpkin pie bites to cool before serving. Optionally, dust with additional pumpkin pie spice for garnish.

Mango Coconut Sorbet

Description: Cool down with this refreshing and tropical mango coconut sorbet, a delightful dairy-free treat perfect for a sunny day.

Cooking Time: 0 minutes

Prep Time: 10 minutes

Freezing Time: 4 hours

Servings: 4

Ingredients:

2 ripe mangoes, peeled and diced

1 can (13.5 oz) coconut milk (full-fat)

1/4 cup honey or maple syrup

1 tablespoon lime juice

Pinch of salt

Fresh mint leaves for garnish (optional)

Nutritional Information (per serving):

Calories: 220

Total Fat: 14g

Saturated Fat: 12g

Sodium: 10mg

Total Carbohydrates: 25g

Dietary Fiber: 2g

Sugars: 21g

Protein: 2g

Preparation Steps:

Blend Mixture: Place diced mangoes, coconut milk, honey or maple syrup, lime juice, and a pinch of salt in a blender. Blend until smooth and creamy.

Freeze: Pour the mixture into a shallow container and freeze for 4 hours, or until firm.

Softening: Once frozen, remove the sorbet from the freezer and let it sit at room temperature for a few minutes to soften slightly.

Serve: Scoop the sorbet into bowls, garnish with fresh mint leaves if desired, and serve immediately.

Berry Crumble Bars

Description: Enjoy the irresistible combination of sweet berries and buttery crumble in these wholesome and satisfying bars, suitable for a quick breakfast or snack.

Cooking Time: 30 minutes

Prep Time: 15 minutes

Servings: 12

Ingredients:

2 cups mixed berries (e.g. strawberries, blueberries, raspberries)

2 tablespoons maple syrup

1 tablespoon cornstarch

1 cup old-fashioned oats

1/2 cup almond flour

1/4 cup coconut sugar

1/2 teaspoon ground cinnamon

1/4 cup coconut oil, melted

1 teaspoon vanilla extract

Pinch of salt

Nutritional Information (per serving):

Calories: 150

Total Fat: 7g

Saturated Fat: 4g

Sodium: 5mg

Total Carbohydrates: 21g

Dietary Fiber: 3g

Sugars: 9g

Protein: 2g

Preparation Steps:

Preheat Oven: Preheat your oven to 350°F (175°C) and line an 8x8-inch baking dish with parchment paper.

Prepare Berry Mixture: In a bowl, toss the mixed berries with maple syrup and cornstarch until well coated. Spread the berry mixture evenly in the bottom of the prepared baking dish.

Prepare Oat Mixture: In another bowl, combine oats, almond flour, coconut sugar, cinnamon, melted coconut oil, vanilla extract, and a pinch of salt. Mix until crumbly.

Assemble Bars: Sprinkle the oat mixture evenly over the berries in the baking dish.

Bake: Bake for 25-30 minutes, or until the topping is golden brown and the berries bubble.

Cool and Slice: Allow the berry crumble bars to cool completely in the baking dish before slicing them into squares.

CHAPTER 12:

SMOOTHIES

Boost your energy and nutrition with a delicious smoothie! This chapter presents quick and easy smoothie recipes perfect for any time of day. From the Green Detox Smoothie to the Creamy Chocolate Avocado Smoothie, these recipes will refresh and revitalize your body, one sip at a time.

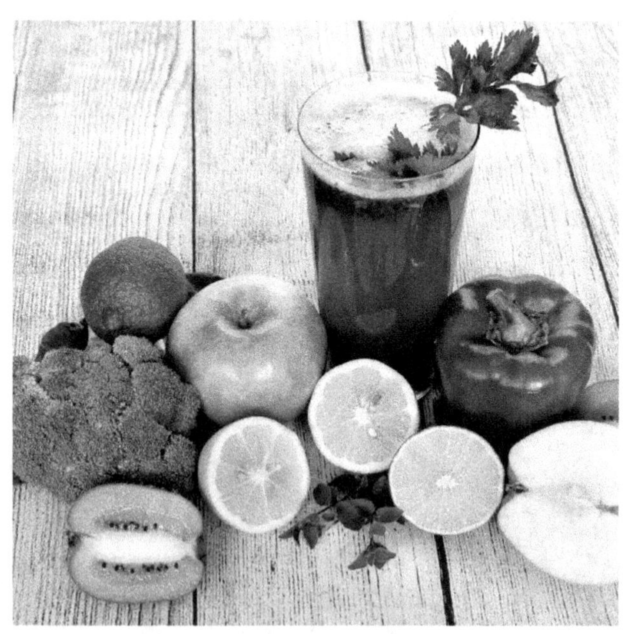

Green Detox Smoothie

Description: Kickstart your day with this refreshing green detox smoothie, packed with nutrient-rich ingredients to cleanse and revitalize your body.

Prep Time: 5 minutes

Servings: 2

Ingredients:

2 cups fresh spinach

1 ripe banana

1 green apple, cored and chopped

1/2 cucumber, chopped

1 tablespoon fresh ginger, grated

1 tablespoon fresh lemon juice

1 cup coconut water or almond milk

Ice cubes (optional)

Nutritional Information (per serving):

Calories: 110

Total Fat: 0.5g

Saturated Fat: 0g

Sodium: 95mg

Total Carbohydrates: 28g

Dietary Fiber: 5g

Sugars: 16g

Protein: 3g

Preparation Steps:

Add Ingredients: Place spinach, banana, green apple, cucumber, ginger, lemon juice, and coconut water or almond milk in a blender.

Blend: Blend until smooth and creamy.

Add Ice (Optional): If desired, add ice cubes and blend again until well incorporated.

Serve: Pour into glasses and enjoy this refreshing green detox smoothie to start your day feeling energized and revitalized.

Berry Blast Smoothie

Description: Satisfy your cravings for something sweet and refreshing with this vibrant berry blast smoothie, bursting with antioxidants and flavor.

Prep Time: 5 minutes

Servings: 2

Ingredients:

1 cup mixed berries (such strawberries, blueberries, and raspberries)

1 ripe banana

1 cup plain Greek yogurt

1 tablespoon honey or maple syrup

1/2 cup almond milk or coconut water

Ice cubes (optional)

Nutritional Information (per serving):

Calories: 160

Total Fat: 1g

Saturated Fat: 0g

Sodium: 45mg

Total Carbohydrates: 32g

Dietary Fiber: 4g

Sugars: 22g

Protein: 8g

Preparation Steps:

Add Ingredients: Place mixed berries, banana, Greek yogurt, honey or maple syrup, and almond milk or coconut water in a blender.

Blend: Blend until smooth and creamy.

Add Ice (Optional): Add ice cubes if desired and blend again until well incorporated.

Serve: Pour into glasses and enjoy this delicious berry blast smoothie as a refreshing snack or breakfast treat.

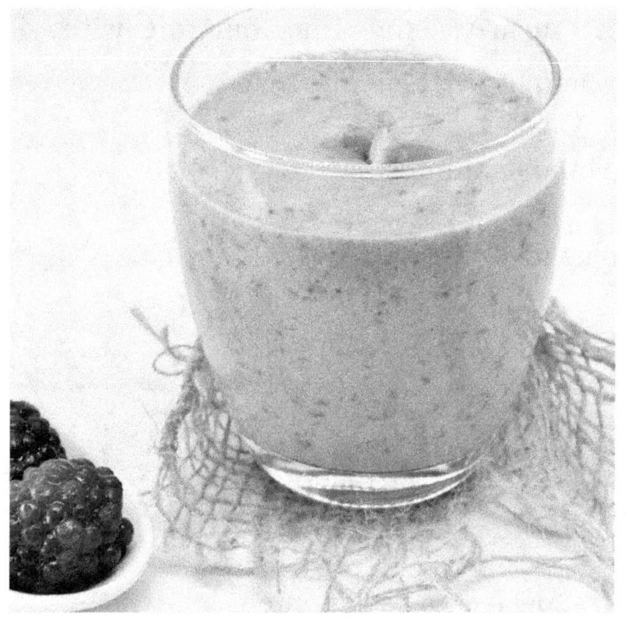

Tropical Turmeric Smoothie

Description: Transport yourself to a tropical paradise with this exotic and anti-inflammatory tropical turmeric smoothie, bursting with vibrant flavors and health benefits.

Prep Time: 5 minutes

Servings: 2

Ingredients:

1 cup pineapple chunks

1 ripe banana

1 orange, peeled and segmented

1/2 teaspoon ground turmeric

1 tablespoon fresh lime juice

1 cup coconut water or pineapple juice

Ice cubes (optional)

Nutritional Information (per serving):

Calories: 130

Total Fat: 0.5g

Saturated Fat: 0g

Sodium: 80mg

Total Carbohydrates: 33g

Dietary Fiber: 4g

Sugars: 21g

Protein: 2g

Preparation Steps:

Add Ingredients: Place pineapple chunks, banana, orange segments, ground turmeric, lime juice, and coconut water or pineapple juice in a blender.

Blend: Blend until smooth and creamy.

Add Ice (Optional): Add ice cubes if desired and blend again until well incorporated.

Serve: Pour into glasses and savor the tropical goodness of this invigorating turmeric smoothie.

Chocolate Avocado Smoothie

Description: Indulge in your chocolate cravings guilt-free with this creamy and decadent chocolate avocado smoothie, packed with healthy fats and antioxidants.

Prep Time: 5 minutes

Servings: 2

Ingredients:

1 ripe avocado

2 tablespoons cocoa powder

2 tablespoons honey or maple syrup

1 cup almond milk or coconut milk

1/2 teaspoon vanilla extract

Ice cubes (optional)

Nutritional Information (per serving):

Calories: 240

Total Fat: 15g

Saturated Fat: 3g

Sodium: 90mg

Total Carbohydrates: 30g

Dietary Fiber: 8g

Sugars: 18g

Protein: 3g

Preparation Steps:

Scoop Avocado: Scoop the ripe avocado flesh into a blender.

Add Ingredients: Add cocoa powder, honey or maple syrup, almond milk or coconut milk, and vanilla extract to the blender.

Blend: Blend until smooth and creamy.

Add Ice (Optional): Add ice cubes if desired and blend again until well incorporated.

Serve: Pour into glasses and indulge in this chocolate avocado smoothie.

Peanut Butter Banana Smoothie

Description: Indulge in the classic combination of creamy peanut butter and sweet bananas with this satisfying and protein-packed smoothie.

Prep Time: 5 minutes

Servings: 2

Ingredients:

2 ripe bananas

2 tablespoons peanut butter

1 cup plain Greek yogurt

1 tablespoon honey or maple syrup

1 cup almond milk or dairy milk

Ice cubes (optional)

Nutritional Information (per serving):

Calories: 280

Total Fat: 10g

Saturated Fat: 2g

Sodium: 150mg

Total Carbohydrates: 38g

Dietary Fiber: 4g

Sugars: 22g

Protein: 14g

Preparation Steps:

Peel Bananas: Peel the bananas and blend them.

Add Ingredients: Add peanut butter, Greek yogurt, honey or maple syrup, and almond milk or dairy milk to the blender.

Blend: Blend until smooth and creamy.

Add Ice (Optional): Add ice cubes if desired and blend again until well incorporated.

Serve: Pour into glasses and enjoy this delicious peanut butter banana smoothie.

Mango Tango Smoothie

Description: Dance to the tropical beat with this vibrant mango tango smoothie, bursting with sunshine and flavor.

Prep Time: 5 minutes

Servings: 2

Ingredients:

2 cups frozen mango chunks

1 ripe banana

1 cup orange juice

1/2 cup plain Greek yogurt

1 tablespoon honey or maple syrup

Ice cubes (optional)

Nutritional Information (per serving):

Calories: 220

Total Fat: 1g

Saturated Fat: 0g

Sodium: 25mg

Total Carbohydrates: 50g

Dietary Fiber: 4g

Sugars: 40g

Protein: 6g

Preparation Steps:

Add Ingredients: Place frozen mango chunks, banana, orange juice, Greek yogurt, and honey or maple syrup in a blender.

Blend: Blend until smooth and creamy.

Add Ice (Optional): Add ice cubes if desired and blend again until well incorporated.

Serve: Pour into glasses and savor the tropical goodness of this mango tango smoothie.

Spinach and Pineapple Smoothie

Description: Get your greens in with this refreshing spinach pineapple smoothie, packed with vitamins and minerals to nourish your body.

Prep Time: 5 minutes

Servings: 2

Ingredients:

2 cups fresh spinach

1 cup frozen pineapple chunks

1 ripe banana

1 cup coconut water or almond milk

1/2 teaspoon grated ginger

Juice of 1/2 lime

Ice cubes (optional)

Nutritional Information (per serving):

Calories: 120

Total Fat: 0.5g

Saturated Fat: 0g

Sodium: 65mg

Total Carbohydrates: 30g

Dietary Fiber: 4g

Sugars: 18g

Protein: 3g

Preparation Steps:

Add Ingredients: Place fresh spinach, frozen pineapple chunks, banana, coconut water or almond milk, grated ginger, and lime juice in a blender.

Blend: Blend until smooth and creamy.

Add Ice (Optional): Add ice cubes if desired and blend again until well incorporated.

Serve: Pour into glasses and enjoy this healthy spinach pineapple smoothie.

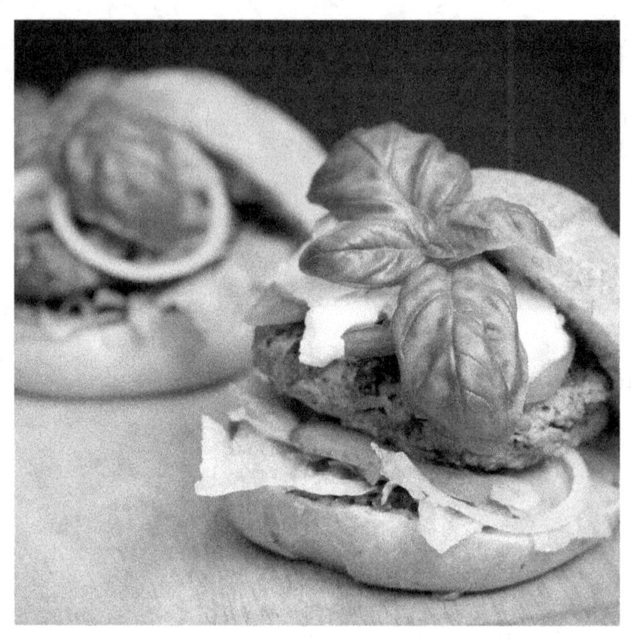

Blueberry Kale Smoothie

Description: Power up your day with this antioxidant-rich blueberry kale smoothie, bursting with vibrant color and nutritional goodness.

Prep Time: 5 minutes

Servings: 2

Ingredients:

1 cup blueberries (fresh or frozen)

1 cup chopped kale leaves (stems removed)

1 ripe banana

1/2 cup plain Greek yogurt

1 tablespoon honey or maple syrup

1 cup almond milk or dairy milk

Ice cubes (optional)

Nutritional Information (per serving):

Calories: 180

Total Fat: 2g

Saturated Fat: 0g

Sodium: 85mg

Total Carbohydrates: 38g

Dietary Fiber: 6g

Sugars: 24g

Protein: 8g

Preparation Steps:

Add Ingredients: Place blueberries, chopped kale leaves, banana, Greek yogurt, honey or maple syrup, and almond milk or dairy milk in a blender.

Blend: Blend until smooth and creamy.

Add Ice (Optional): Add ice cubes if desired and blend again until well incorporated.

Serve: Pour into glasses and enjoy this nourishing blueberry kale smoothie.

Orange Creamsicle Smoothie

Description: Indulge in the nostalgic flavors of a classic creamsicle with this delightful and refreshing orange creamsicle smoothie, a must-have for brightening up your day.

Prep Time: 5 minutes

Servings: 2

Ingredients:

2 large oranges, peeled and segmented

1 ripe banana

1 cup plain Greek yogurt

1 tablespoon honey or maple syrup

1/2 teaspoon vanilla extract

Ice cubes (optional)

Nutritional Information (per serving):

Calories: 180

Total Fat: 0.5g

Saturated Fat: 0g

Sodium: 50mg

Total Carbohydrates: 35g

Dietary Fiber: 3g

Sugars: 25g

Protein: 11g

Preparation Steps:

Add Ingredients: Place orange segments, banana, Greek yogurt, honey or maple syrup, and vanilla extract in a blender.

Blend: Blend until smooth and creamy.

Add Ice (Optional): Add ice cubes if desired and blend again until well incorporated.

Serve: Pour into glasses and enjoy the creamy and tangy goodness of this orange creamsicle smoothie.

Peachy Keen Smoothie

Description: Enjoy a creamy and luscious smoothie packed with ripe peach flavor this summer.

Prep Time: 5 minutes

Servings: 2

Ingredients:

2 ripe peaches, pitted and chopped

1 ripe banana

1 cup coconut water or almond milk

1/2 cup plain Greek yogurt

1 tablespoon honey or maple syrup

Ice cubes (optional)

Nutritional Information (per serving):

Calories: 180

Total Fat: 1g

Saturated Fat: 0g

Sodium: 45mg

Total Carbohydrates: 38g

Dietary Fiber: 4g

Sugars: 30g

Protein: 8g

Preparation Steps:

Add Ingredients: Place chopped peaches, banana, coconut water or almond milk, Greek yogurt, and honey or maple syrup in a blender.

Blend: Blend until smooth and creamy.

Add Ice (Optional): Add ice cubes if desired and blend again until well incorporated.

Serve: Pour into glasses and enjoy the juicy and refreshing flavor of this Peachy Keen smoothie.

CONCLUSIONS

Congratulations on completing this comprehensive cookbook! You now possess a wealth of knowledge and tools to navigate life without a gallbladder with confidence. Remember, this journey is about more than just recipes – it's about taking control of your digestive health and empowering yourself through knowledge and self-care.

As you continue on this path, recall the key takeaways from this book:

Understanding the gallbladder's role in digestion

Modifying your diet to accommodate your body's new needs

Preparing delicious and nutritious meals

Planning meals and shopping with ease

Gaining confidence in your ability to manage your digestive health

Remember, every meal is an opportunity to nourish your body and spirit. Embrace the flavors, cherish the experiences, and celebrate your progress toward a happier, healthier you.

Thank you for joining me on this journey. Happy cooking and happy healing!

BONUS SECTION

30-Day Meal Plan Overview

Welcome to your 30-day meal plan! This structured program offers a variety of delicious and nutritious recipes to support your digestive health. Feel free to adjust the plan to suit your preferences and schedule.

Using the Meal Plan:

Understand the table structure: Day, Breakfast, Snack 1, Lunch, Snack 2, Dinner, and Dessert.

Mix and match recipes based on your preferences and schedule.

Consult your doctor to verify suitable meal combinations.

Prep ingredients ahead to save time.

Drink plenty of water and enjoy herbal teas or infused waters.

Eat slowly, savor each bite, and aim for balanced meals with protein, healthy fats, and fiber-rich carbs.

Incorporate gentle exercise, like walking or yoga, into your daily routine.

Important Reminders:

Meet your nutritional needs by including a variety of foods.

Consult your doctor about specific dietary restrictions or health conditions.

Adjust portion sizes based on hunger and activity level.

Store leftovers properly and reheat them thoroughly.

Keep your kitchen clean and organized.

Substitute ingredients based on availability or taste preferences.

Enjoy your meal plan and happy cooking!

Shopping List Overview

Welcome to your comprehensive shopping list! This organized guide is designed to make your grocery trips efficient and stress-free, ensuring you have all the ingredients needed for a month of delicious, gallbladder-friendly meals.

How to Use the Shopping List:

Organized by categories: Produce, Proteins, Dairy, and more, to navigate the store with ease.

Break down by weeks: Shop weekly for fresh ingredients, if preferred.

Check your pantry: Before shopping, avoid unnecessary purchases and stay within budget.

Adjust quantities: Based on household size, dietary needs, and personal consumption.

Tips for Successful Shopping:

Review meal plan and shopping list: Before heading out, to avoid missing items.

Choose seasonal produce: Fresh, tasty, and affordable.

Store groceries properly: Use airtight containers and appropriate fridge sections.

Substitutions are okay: If an ingredient is unavailable, find an alternative.

Prepare and freeze: Larger quantities of recipes for later use.

Use up versatile ingredients: Plan to use quinoa, beans, and other multi-recipe ingredients throughout the week.

Freeze wilting produce: Berries, bananas, and leafy greens can be frozen for later use.

Happy shopping!